iCanSir!

How a Breakthrough Mind-Body Technology
called Emotional Archaeology
can help you find hope and connection
in the cancer experience...

No Matter What!

previously released as
Jumper Cables for the Healing Soul
How to Embrace the Moment, Celebrate the Past, and Welcome
the Future With Gratitude, Grit and Grace...No Matter What!

By George P. Kansas

Copyright George P. Kansas, 2011, Delmar, New York

ISBN 978-0-9763573-3-9 Hardcover
ISBN 978-0-9763573-4-6 Ebook
ISBN 978-0-9763573-5-3 Softcover

Journeypress

iCanSir!

iCanSir!

A thought before we begin.

You are the captain of your dream
Your friends and family are its crew.
Your predecessors; its benefactors
Your progeny; its beneficiaries
And the world; its commission

Its hull was fashioned from the character of your ancestors
Enthusiasm, Insight and Faith are its sails
Its masts are hewn from Courage
Its ropes and lines; spun from Experience
Its rudder; forged from Pain

When your dream lists, your crew helps to right it
When you stagger from the helm, your crew takes the wheel
When it takes on ballast, you bail and purge together
All know its purpose, so its compass is always true

Arm in arm, there is no sea we cannot cross,
No storm we cannot weather,
No maelstrom we cannot navigate;
On our cosmopolitan journey!

You are the captain of your dream.
Your dream awaits.
Welcome aboard!

iCanSir!

Dedications

This book is dedicated to my kids, Peter and Tessa, my entire loving family, Drs. Peter Burkart and Rachel Grimm, and the doctors, nurses and staff of the Cancer and Blood Disorders Center on D4E at Albany Medical Center Hospital. I literally wouldn't have been able to finish this book without each and every one of you!

Expressions of Gratitude

Thank you, my wonderful children, Peter and Tessa. You awe me - non-stop - every single day! Thank you, Maria, for taking care of the kids and bringing me coffee and doughnuts (and chicken Marsala, and bacon sandwiches, and sausage, peppers and onions!). Thank you Elaine for reminding me that I had written the book on getting through a marathon[1] and – reading it myself - that's exactly what I did! Thank you, Dad, for our walk down New Scotland Ave. Like Mom, you eased my fears and didn't even know it. It meant the world to me.

Thank you to Dr. Peter T. Burkart, MD for saving my life. You've helped so many people live to serve their purpose. In doing so, you serve a wonderful purpose of your own. Mine can continue to be served because of your experience, compassion and judgment. I intend to be grateful for your skills for a very, very long time!

Thank you to Dr. Rachel Grimm, MD. You don't know how much I looked forward to our chats in the morning. You have a great attitude and you gave me permission to have mine!

Thank you to the whole gang of angels at D4E and NYOH. You're all awesome!

---

[1] For more information about this wonderful tool for the athletes in your life, please visit; www.georgepkansas.com

iCanSir!

To all you folks out there who, like I used to, give blood so that people like me can stay alive a bit longer exactly when we need to!

To all my friends, thankfully too many to list, and just plain nice people who sent me cards, brought me food or just sat there as I slept. I am grateful. Deeply, deeply so.

To my dear friend Immaculée Ilibagiza; your grace and kindness means so much to me. I am so very grateful to you for your encouragement and assistance with this book. I'm even more so to God for sparing you so that you could teach the world about the power of forgiveness!

To my editor, Claire 'Denny' Hughes: I am grateful for your firm guidance and more so for the grace with which you wielded it.

iCanSir!

Table of Contents

iCanSir!

Prologue

I almost died. Then I woke up.

This is what I learned.

iCanSir!

Forward

Have you ever been unsure of yourself or your future? Have you ever been scared? Really scared? What about confused? Ever been confused?

Of course, right? Of course.

Have you ever feared death? Ever been so afraid to die or so afraid that you might die that you felt aware of panic overcoming you? Have you feared other things that have had the same effect on you? Ever felt this fear affect your ability to truly live?

Maybe you know what's up. Maybe not. Maybe you're waiting for the other shoe to drop. Maybe you're just confused. Maybe you're waiting for test results and you fear the unknown. Perhaps you're wallowing in a profound depression. Perhaps you're just lost. Drifting amidst the living, feeling like a purposeless soul with no direction, no passions to speak of and no vocabulary with which to describe your helplessness.

I know the feeling.

Sometimes you just don't know what to think. It can be scary, huh? I think that anyone who's struggled with either a disease like cancer or something else that threatens - in a very big way - the everyday way in which we approach our lives, can appreciate how disorienting such an experience can be. Many have been there. Far too many.

Me too. We've all been there to a certain degree at some point. It's the human condition. Having gone through it myself, felt those fears many times personally, I've had the combined blessings of - on the one hand - having the skills, training and experience to observe, analyze and articulate the lessons from these challenges and - on the other hand - having survived them to tell the tale. Along the way, having applied those skills, made those observations, sought the answers, I figured out a way to alleviate some of the deep distress that can come with some of these experiences.

Stumbled upon it might be a better way to put it than "figured it out". Upon stumbling, however, I discovered a way to turn fear into the actual constructive energy necessary for healing, growth and, well, love. I want so badly for you to know this, that I wrote this book for you. I've committed my professional life to sharing the messages in this book with audiences since I first could venture out of my house upon my recovery.

Most of this particular set of inspirations came during an ordeal with Leukemia that I experienced at forty. Having shared the ideas with all sorts of people, however, I've come to understand that it doesn't have to be cancer you're dealing with in order to benefit from these ideas. They apply to break-ups, career changes, bad relationships, parenting... you name it. Why? Because fear impacts all of us and potentially in all situations. Managing that fear is important.

There are a handful of ideas I'm going to share with you in this book. The ideas are essentially centuries old but until my cancer experience, I had never heard them put quite this way. When I experienced this understanding, suddenly I was able to articulate these ideas a bit differently than I had heard them before. Specifically, I understand them now as they related to health and how we manifest healing and balance in our lives. The first idea is spelled out in this forward so I won't mention it in this paragraph.

For the sake of giving you a heads up on what you'll encounter further along, and sort of as a primer for how to best use this book, I'll tell you a bit more about what you'll see later on. In subsequent chapters I'll explain how I came to understand that no matter what you're dealing with, there's stuff to find humor in, stuff to be grateful for, stuff to forgive yourself and others for and how important all of that is. I'll tell you how I came to understand that the 'cancer was me'.

iCanSir!

I'll explain what the heck that means and why I was glad I made that realization. No one had ever explained it that way, I just sort of figured it out and I'm pretty sure it saved my life.

I'll show you how, whether you're well or unwell, that idea can change your life. I'll also explain how I came to understand that maybe it's time we change the metaphor of healing from one of war to one of peace. You'll read about my experience with both, and how I'm certain the use of a peaceful, forgiving method of healing was the more beneficial and helpful of the two. I'll get into how to meditate and use that skill to become mindful of the answers you're seeking. I'll help you figure out the differences among what you want to do, what you have to do and what you were born to do. And finally, you'll get started on establishing habits that will help you make the most of the rest of your life. It's a tall order but I'm confident that if you join me for this part of the journey, you'll be proud you did.

At forty years old, my first day in the hospital one day in February, was also the first day I was directly confronted with the fear of impending, imminent personal mortality. Finding out I was sick and needed medical attention would have been one thing, but discovering that this illness could be deadly as well and becoming aware of these ideas on the same weekend was kind of a heavy trip. On the other hand, having to deal with the big idea of mortality in a compressed time frame forced me to keep my focus. On the whole, I'm grateful that I had to get my arms around both illness as well as death at the same time. I figure that all of life isn't going to be happy, happy. But I've always tried to look at it the right way. When I've done that, I've noticed I could feel the pain and be grateful anyway.

During these times, inspirations have reliably swept over me. As you will read, during my cancer experience - true to form - the universe struck me with a series of inspirations.

The first of these key ideas – if we can get enough people to embrace – will change the world. I didn't make it up. My illness just made me aware of it.

That idea is this:

Our adversities may be different.
They don't separate us.

While I first sat in my bed as a newly admitted patient, suddenly I had peace and quiet. An interesting respite from a hectic and busy life of accomplishment. What would have ordinarily driven me crazy - a complete lack of frenetic activity around me - suddenly felt oddly reassuring. Suddenly I had time to meditate. My caregivers were insisting on my rest and non-disturbance. It was as if the universe was telling me (more like scolding me) "Hey you, Mr. Get it Done, Now. Take a moment and reflect!"

I first invested that time simply absorbing my situation. Literally looking around my room. Noticing the window view, the television and video cassette recorder. The screens and draw curtains for privacy. The bathroom, the chairs for visitors, the radiator/air conditioning unit. Finally, I took in the bed. What was to become my home for nearly a month. My tiny little universe had shrunken even smaller. I thought, Wow, you know? If you take everybody and stick them in a bed, tethered to a transfusion machine, bedridden and completely dependent upon the care and support of others, we're all pretty much the same. Strip away the "stuff" and "jobs" and pretty quickly we become very, very similar. Very little actually separates us. Suddenly, far more things about me became exactly the same as most of the things about the other people around me. My fellow hospital mates. My new neighborhood.

As I thought about that idea and let it sink in, I became very aware of how much time and energy we spend in identifying ways to separate ourselves from one another. From the color of our skin (just a few cells thick) to the number of commas on our bank statement (just a few drops of ink), many of the ways we fabricate to separate ourselves from one another became suddenly obvious to me.

As I thought about how dependence linked me to everyone else in the hospital, I realized how – absent the perspective of involuntary dependence – we concentrate, on a day-to-day basis, more on how we are different from most other people. What set me apart? What made me unique and special? I realized that I wasn't really alone in that mentality. I had been thinking like that despite the benefit of a lot of experiences having taught me the value of interdependence, and the importance of a balance among self-reliance and community. I realized that if I had once again become caught up in that, by comparison, generally we must all lean quite far toward the "separation" end of the spectrum. That simply must not be healthy.

Rather than invest that energy in figuring out how we're connected, we simply focus on what separates us. And it's killing us. It's probably easier to do in the short run, but that doesn't mean it's good for us. I mean, if you think about it, as I thought about it, if you put all of us in hospital beds, stripped us of our strength and vitality, make us all helpless and dependent on others to care for us, we'd all be the same then wouldn't we? So why should the addition of a little health and vitality and interdependence change things so dramatically? I don't think it should. When I was lying in bed, I figured it was a shame that we let it.

I had a rare form of cancer. It could have been a different type of cancer. It could have been any number of things. You may have had a severe injury. You may feel depressed. You actually may be depressed. You may be recovering from a dependency. You may be scared. You may be drifting in limbo. You may be suffering terribly. You may be broke. You may be involved in a relationship that is, it is clear to everyone but you, not healthy for you. You may be caring for someone who is unable to take care of themselves. You may feel incredibly despondent. You may feel absolutely without cause or purpose.

The end result is while I'm writing this, I can't know what you're going through. Each of us has our own challenges. But the fact that those challenges differ, doesn't mean that we don't share something.

The fact that we're each of us unique,
doesn't mean that we're not all of us connected.

It could be the suffering that connects us. It could be the celebration. I don't know for sure. I just know we're connected by something. I call it energy. In my speeches – audiences for which are as diverse as America itself – I refer to it as the energy of the universe. I've heard it called lots of things. I've even heard it called God. If it is God, I think that's the best definition of God I've heard yet; the universal energy that animates and connects all of us. Getting hung up on what words we use to describe it, however, is part of our problem. For millennia, we've started wars over what we call and how we interpret this energy. The bottom line is that right now, you're at a place where you're open to the idea that what we call it is far less important than putting it to work for you! You just wouldn't be reading this right now if that weren't so.

No matter what we call it, this energy connects us. Quantum physicists tell us that this energy not only connects us but also comprises us and every other thing. Everything in the universe is made up of energy. Each "particle" of energy vibrates at a certain frequency. The frequency at which it's vibrating and the frequency at which we're vibrating will determine how we perceive it. Since everything is made of this same energy, including the "stuff" that "separates" us, then we must be connected in some way to everyone and everything. That's the quantum physics lesson for this chapter. You don't have to understand this to believe it. Energy connects us. All of us.

Why I bring this idea of connection up at this point is because no matter what the specific challenges you may be dealing with, this information will work for you. It will work for you because it worked for me and has worked for thousands of people whom I've had the honor of working with or the pleasure of reading about. My own experience confirms this. Since we have more in common than not, it will work for you too. No matter who you are, or what your situation. Put it to work and it will work!

So while technically this may be considered a "cancer book" (whatever that is or is supposed to be), it's really an "any type of adversity that affects one's health" book. And when I say "health" I'm referring, of course, to physical health, yes, but I'm also referring to emotional and even spiritual health. Which is to say that really, this is an "anything you could possibly be experiencing" type book.

I don't pretend to know all the answers. I am not even sure I am asking the appropriate questions half of the time. I think that if you are looking at these words right now, either you think you may, or someone you know thinks you may, be able to relate to and benefit from what I have to say here.

At the time I started writing this book, my leukemia was a cancer of the blood and bone marrow (the part of your body which is responsible for making new blood). This leukemia inhibited an important biological process in my body that biologists and doctors call hematopoesis or new blood production.

By the time this book was finished, that cancer had left my body. The leukemia I was diagnosed with proved itself to be manageable. I am fortunate. As I write this, I am in remission. Although I've learned that things can change in a moment, currently things look good. A year ago and a year out from my first treatment, my doctors told me I'd never have a "normal" hemoglobin level or a "normal" immune system. Today, as I polish the words for this introductory chapter, my

iCanSir!

hemoglobin level is that of a performance athlete and my immune cell counts are in the "normal" range.   For now, I live to fight the proverbial good fight another day.

Whether I have or had cancer, however, is not as important as what I'm about to tell you. What's critical for you to understand is this:

> The ideas I am going to discuss with you in this book, all stem from a series of experiences I had <u>before</u> I found out what my diagnosis was.

> This is important because at the time these ideas came to me, I was certain in my belief that my death was imminent.

I <u>thought</u> what I had was worse than the leukemia I eventually was told I <u>actually</u> had. Reading this now, that distinction may not make that much difference to you. I understand that. I make the point, however, because it makes the inspirations of which I became mindful more credible. This material doesn't stem from a positive attitude derived from the good news of the possibility of a favorable outcome or remission. This information was valid and inspirational when I thought that news would never come. These ideas came to me when I thought - <u>as I imagine many of you might as you're reading this right now</u> – that such news might never be mine to receive.

Which means that I'm certain that the same information will be helpful to you regardless of what the doctors or your advisors are telling you about how the future might look for you.

<u>It means that no matter what you're facing, no matter what your diagnosis is, no matter what your "official" prognosis is, I'm going to encourage you from the very center of my soul to experiment with the information contained in this book.</u>

It will help you deal with what you're dealing with. It will make you a better, more receptive, more participative patient or caregiver. And don't tell your doctors this but it will even help you help your doctors to be better doctors!

My experience with audiences since my cancer has proven to me that it most certainly will help regardless of what step along the path you find yourself today.

The information that came to me in those moments – the information that you'll leave this book knowing - was dramatic, incredibly liberating and completely affirming. I want – in the most intense way – for all people to know the kind of clarity I knew that evening. People with cancer. People without cancer. People with children. People without children. People with careers. People without careers. All people.

On February 6, 2005, as I pondered my own death, and the days subsequent to that, I had the presence of mind to journal it carefully. I'm glad I did because since then, armed with this detailed information, I have helped hundreds of people. With this book I hope to leverage that to thousands and even hundreds of thousands of people. Maybe even millions! That's what I was born to do.

This is the story of a brief period of my life, which includes my first experiences with a serious illness of my own, and the resulting lessons that I gleaned from it. As you must know from your own experiences, it was a hard, painful journey. As a result, some of the language I use might be a bit raw for some people. I offer no apology. Most of the survivors I've worked with appreciate the candor. They usually tell me that it gives them permission to express some of the raw emotions they feel. Sometimes the "vocabulary of survivorship", as I call it, is peaceful, sweet and touching. Sometimes it's just as violent, ugly and merciless as the disease or negativity you're encountering.

✗ iCanSir!

I hope that you don't let the particular language distract you from the intention. My intention is for these ideas to help you maintain perspective. My intention is for that to be true no matter how much of life remains. We have no idea – none of us – how much that is. Whether we're healthy or not, none of us knows. I hope that such perspective may help you to live a life that is closer to the one you may envision for yourself in the quiet, true moments of your mind. I truly wish that for you.

I believe that if more of the world could listen to the honest sound of their true self,

if we could see a clearer vision of who we truly are,

if we could feel that perfect feeling deep down inside ourselves, we would be able to manage our suffering much more effectively.

We might even reduce it a bit.

We might even know peace.

Wouldn't that be so very nice?

Chapter One
"Always…"

While preparing this manuscript, I read a lot about the ancient battle of Thermopylae (in ancient Greece). Maybe it's my Spartan heritage, but my interest coincides with the recent release of a movie depicting the legendary and epic battle. According to historians and Greek lore, at this pivotal battle a relatively small force of 300 Spartans led a group of a few thousand other Greeks to delay the progress across Europe of as many as 600,000 soldiers fighting for the Persian Empire. Many historians credit this battle as having significantly shaped the course of history and paved the way for the further development of western civilization.

Never having been a real history buff, it was difficult for me to get my head around a lot of the references I uncovered in my reading. Fortunately, the books I've been reading have included lots and lots of background information relative to the state of the world in the decades both before and after this pivotal battle. As much as the story of the battle itself, it is this background information that enabled me to understand a little better the true impact of this event. The context, you see, is what has made all the difference.

Likewise, in order to really get what I'm going to convey in this book – and I really want you to get what I'm going to convey – it will help you to have a bit of my background. As with most big ideas, the context will make a difference. If you have an understanding of a series of strange events, you'll appreciate the impact of the inspirations that have come to me as a result of them. If you appreciate them, you'll apply them. If you apply them, your life will improve.

One of the biggest events in my life was the death of my mom. It was a heavy trip to say the least. To get the full effect of that experience and why and how I was poised as I was to receive the full impact of this event, I'll give you a little of the back story behind the back story.

In 1995 I was blessed with the sole legal responsibility of caring for my two children, Peter and Tessa. These two gifts from the universe are the center of things for me. My responsibility to them has shaped my decisions for most of my adult life but most especially for the past 13 years. Honestly, this will probably always be so to a certain degree. Why this is important to my mom's death is because my mother played a critical role in my being able to deal with the many challenges of single parenthood. As I worked during those first couple of years as a single dad, my mother helped me with much of the details of day-to-day child rearing. Transitioning from a practicing attorney and consultant with three offices to a stay-at-home dad working from a home office, was three full-time jobs rolled into one! In short, I couldn't have done it without the support of my whole family. My mom, however, was the key player, without a doubt. On top of the already healthy foundation she had given me as a great role model, my mom undertook many a day's care giving, especially of my little daughter.

Fast-forward five years or so. Peter was ten, almost eleven and Tessa was six, almost seven. My mother was diagnosed with cancer. What started as a tiny spot on her pancreas rapidly worsened. Now, you know what an unpleasant disease cancer can be. I'm sure there is not a particularly "worse" kind of cancer. Having said that, my mom's cancer experience was characterized by severe pain, few - if any - encouraging moments and an overall sense of decline with very little relief from what appeared to be an inevitable and painful death. Now, I'm an optimist and am highly skilled at finding the silver lining. It was difficult to find in those moments. Most of the lessons I gleaned from this experience, I gleaned, after my mom's death. You see moms are moms always, not just while they're alive!

As trying as those last six months were, they were punctuated by some pretty amazing and deep connections. My sisters and I had taken a lot of time off and incurred a lot of personal debt in order to be able to take care of my mom while she was at home. As difficult as it was to do, this allowed for some great memories to be created. Two favorites stand out. The first is a little light moment that I was able to share with my mother with hardly a word being spoken. One afternoon, I was hanging out with Mom in my childhood home. She on the couch and me on the arm-chair. Off the top of my head, I thought to ask if she'd like a shampoo. This isn't something I'd ever done for her nor would it be something I would have ordinarily even thought of. With a big smile she said that would be nice. I got a big bowl and a pitcher of hot water, a couple of towels and a bottle of my mom's shampoo.

After preparing the area with towels for the inevitable spillage I began by simply pouring some warm water slowly over the back of Mom's head as she leaned over the bowl which I had set up on the table at the side of the couch. Once her hair was wet I gently lathered in the shampoo and gently massaged my mom's scalp. I could feel her shrinking, once strong, muscles relaxing underneath my strong hands. She didn't have to say a word. I could tell that although this was something she would have never asked me to do, she was enjoying this moment. It was a rare moment between my mom and I.

How many times had she bathed me? How many times had she scrubbed my filthy body of the dirt my hyperactive antics and embedded upon me as a wild kid? What a handful I must have been! Yet she handled it. Now, as her frail little body slowly gave way to time and cancer, I returned the favor. What a tiny little thing to be able to do for her, but it gave me such great joy.

The second big moment for us would be the last. Over the months Mom gradually became so weak that walking up the stairs was a major effort. One that it was decided we'd better save for bathing since everything else was really available on the ground floor. Everything, that is, but a bed. So, we got a hospital bed and put in smack in the middle of the family room! How's that for service?

One day in January, I sat on the edge of that bed while Mom lay there. My dad and my two sisters stood nearby. Mom had become weaker still, with just moments of lucid time each day. We were upset. For the first time since my high school graduation, it was just my sisters and I and my parents in our home. No spouses, no children, just the five of us.

My mom had struggled to rid her body of pancreatic cancer for five months. During that time she'd suffered all manner of excruciating pain, loss of motor function, hallucinations and difficulty breathing. Like this day, there were times when she'd barely be conscious and then for only minutes in a day. There were times when she was conscious that I secretly wished she wasn't just so that she wouldn't have to endure the mind bending pain the cancer's pressure on her nerve endings were causing her.

But on this day – what was to be her last full day - she was lucid. She was clearly having trouble staying awake and her breathing was labored but she was aware. She was mindful of my father at her side and her children at her feet (literally). We did most of the talking. She did a lot of nodding. Her breathing was labored but occasionally she'd deliberately take an extra deep breath so that she could wheeze a response to a particular point in the conversation. She was trying so hard for our sake. I remember being aware that these were our last moments with Mom. I was also aware that I was aware. It was intense.

A lot of the talk was meant to comfort my mom. To let her know we were there and we were willing to do anything for her. Anything to ease her burden. Anything to ease her pain. When she was well, my sisters and I had usually let her know that we were glad and grateful to have had such a great mom. My dad had always made it clear that he was very much in love with my mom. Flowers, nice gifts, trips, etc. We were a pretty tight family. With all of our faults, failing to express and demonstrate loving emotions didn't seem to be one of them.

Despite that, I had always wanted to – when the time came – let her know "one last time" that she'd done a great job as a mom and, for what it was worth from my point of view, a wife. I wanted to let her know how deeply impressed I had always been by her. I wanted to let her know how proud I was to be her son. That day, at her bedside, I tried to do that.

After choking out the most difficult compliments I would ever pay, I got up and went into an adjoining room. My sisters followed me, leaving my father and mother to be by themselves for a moment. They could tell I needed some comforting. By the time we made it into the other room, I was crying. My sisters asked what in particular was upsetting me. They hadn't seen me cry over mom's illness yet. I guess they wondered what finally tipped the scales. I told them that I felt the need to tell her more. I felt the need to tell her that I was proud of her for having done such a great job. To tell her that I was awed by the fight she'd put up. That she'd taught us all she needed to teach us. That we'd be good parents and good siblings and continue to be good children to Dad. I guess I just wanted to let her know that her work was done and from our point of view, done very well.

My sisters insisted I do just that. "If you don't" they urged, "you'll always wish you had." So, I took a few deep breaths, settled down and did just that.

We went back into our family room (great name for a room when you think about it), just the five of us again. I explained to Mom that I had to say it again. I told her that I felt she needed to know that she'd done such a wonderful job as a mother. I explained that she had taught us all that we needed to know to take it from here. That she needn't worry about us any longer. That we'd be fine.

She looked with her wise, deep brown eyes into mine. She looked at me with neither confidence and certainty nor fear and trepidation. She looked at me with a sad peace. Sadness, I think, not relating to her death necessarily but rather to the many days we would not invest together as a result of it. I was sad for the same reason.

Her gaze pierced me to my very soul. She drew her labored breath. She said, "Take care of your daughter!" I drew a short breath and – although with difficulty - I held my composure. I was so deeply touched by her maternal concern for my little baby girl. "Take care of your son!" Again, it was all I could do to hold myself together.

"Of course," I said. "I'll take care of the kids" I assured her. "Don't worry about anything, I'll take care of everyone." I was reassuring myself as well. It may have been bravado, but it kept me together for a few seconds longer. I was sincere, though, in my assertion. I was deriving confidence from her power!

"I want to ask you just one favor." I asked, somehow knowing this would be the last I'd ever speak with the woman who'd borne me, changed my diapers, nourished me, body and soul. The woman who'd invested half her life in nurturing mine was dying and I knew it. At the same time, she had such a knowing look in her eyes. Such a knowing demeanor about her. As if she knew exactly where she was going and when and how and why.

Her eyes never wavered from mine and my gaze would not falter either. "Keep an eye on us?" I asked.

She blinked with the most precious, sweet slowness as she drew yet another breath. I could almost feel the pain she was enduring as each breath crowded her internal organs, tumors and nerves and yet, the pain seemed to be leaving her, or perhaps guiding her. Her calm and peacefulness humbled me. My attention was rapt.

Again her deep, knowing eyes pierced mine. She drew me ever so gently toward her so that my ear was just an inch away from her lips. "Always…" she whispered as she slowly exhaled her shallow breath. I lifted my head to look her in her eyes. She had the sweetest, most subtle, most reassuring smile on her face. It was a different smile than the one I had grown up with. It was her "cancer smile" as I'd grown to think of it. It was the smile that she was capable of while enduring pain that would cripple a weaker person. Harder for her to deliver but just as wonderful for me to behold. What a doll she was to do and say that. Such a good mother, right to the very end.

It struck me that such a deep, strong and piercing message could come from the shallow breath of such a weakened body. It struck me that, in the final analysis, there was nothing weak about my mother in that moment. In fact, the strength of the universe was hers in the very moment she imparted that secret unto me. The strength of the gods of Olympus itself was hers, mine and ours together.

In that moment, in that tiny word, in that wisp of a breath and that deep gaze, my fear of death was vanquished. "Always!"

Not uttering another word out of fear of tarnishing this perfectly executed goodbye, I kissed my mother on the cheek and forehead and patted her hand ever so gently. My goodbye to my mother had been, in my mind, perfect.

I said goodbye to my dad and my sisters and I walked out through the garage. I remember being so very mindful of the fact that my Mother's body would die that night. I had carried on my last conversation with my Mother's physical presence. I also knew in my bones, however, that I would have many more with her in my consciousness. She had promised me after all. "Always!"

I am as certain as I can be that, in that moment, my Mother had a very clear sense of what was awaiting her. In fact, I'd go so far as to say that she knew exactly what was happening and how and why. I've got a feeling she pretty much had all the answers in that moment.

I mentioned context. I've explained this to you for two reasons. The first reason is that it has proven to really reach people as a very inspiring story about the kind of peace we're capable of knowing in our last hours. That might bring you some peace of your own no matter what the immediate future may look like for you because – after all – none of us know exactly when "our time" will be. It certainly has given me an incredible amount of peace.

The second reason is really to give you a big piece of background so that you'll understand where I was coming from as the additional stories you're about to read unfold.

This one word and, of course, the gaze that had accompanied it, transformed my entire outlook on death. It affected how I looked at mortality, the condition of my soul, how death might greet me, how I might - from then on - approach my life. As you read this book, my hope is that it will have an effect on the way you approach your life too. Your illness, your wellness, your relationships, the whole package. Keep this in mind as you read on.

As I encountered serious illness in my own life, this is the context with which my experience was surrounded.

"Always!"

Has a nice ring to it!

§ iCanSir!

Chapter Two
"You should be unconscious!"

For months, my heart pounded at the slightest exertion. Even the deepest breathing wasn't satisfying my body's need for vital oxygen. I was actually hearing my heartbeat in my ear drums - literally, all of the time. I was panting like a dog. Taking off my clothes to crawl into bed made my heart scream at me. And I didn't know why.

The winter before, while skiing in the Wasatch Mountains of Utah with my father, I had experienced my first bout with altitude sickness. This despite the fact that I'd been active at high altitudes all over the world without ever having had a problem since I'd been ten years old. Altitude sickness affects people in different ways. The most common symptoms are shortness of breath, chest pain, weakness, nausea and dizziness. I experienced all of them.

I'd had a physical exam around my birthday the previous summer that showed no signs of any problem. Of course, the prescription for my annual complete blood count and cholesterol check remained unfulfilled because I didn't want to hear anyone tell me that I had to watch my cholesterol. I know, I know. Stupid! Just wait, it gets worse. Much worse. My behavior over the subsequent 12 months redefined "stupid".

Later that year, in spring, I had experienced some shortness of breath while running around the neighborhood. During the next summer, while playing on the beach on Cape Cod with my kids and nephews, I noticed I would get out of breath, tiring very quickly and experiencing the sensation of my heart pounding so hard that I could hear it in my ear drums. This is called palpitation. Since then – after months of gradually worsening palpitation - I had been "toughing it out", chocking it up to having hit my fortieth year and being "out of shape". In my bones, I knew it wasn't so, but denial is a powerful thing.

iCanSir!

As if those hints weren't direct enough, my then new boutique record label – Yodeling Loon Records - was working on a record with a group of great local musicians. My "loons" as I called them. We'd been working into the wee hours for weeks in an effort to get a CD finished in time for a pre-Christmas release. As it turned out we just couldn't pull it off between all the different musicians' schedules and available studio time. Coming home from the studio at 3 a.m. a couple of nights a week hadn't been out of the ordinary for me. I was really pushing it.

Each morning I would wake up and the kids would have to hoist me out of bed. "C'mon dad, you've got to get up and make our lunches. You've got to wake up." They'd admonish me as they – literally – dragged my exhausted butt out of bed. I just thought this was what it meant to burn the candle at both ends. I knew I had to slow down but I was having so much fun tackling all of these projects that were important to me.

The straw that broke the camel's back, however, came on January 30, 2005 when my kids, my sister, my nephews, my dad and my step-mother went skiing. Now, we are usually an aggressive bunch on the slopes. We ski as we live. With gusto! After skiing for about 6 hours we were ready to call it a day. Usually for the last few runs of the day I'll open it up and let my skis really run. I'll go as fast as I can in a real down-hill style after I've let the family get down the mountain a bit ahead of me. As I whizzed past the kids my heart became louder and louder in my ears.

Finally, I stopped. My chest felt like it was on fire. The pain in my heart and lungs was excruciating. I doubled over. Barely standing. I was reeling in pain. My chest was tightening by the second, my heart was pounding and my lungs felt as though flame had engulfed them. Each breath drew in a searing heat that scorched my insides. I didn't know what was going on. I assumed I was having a heart attack.

♀ iCanSir!

My dad and sister – both physicians – were concerned (needless to say). After a few minutes of sucking wind (as we used to call it at football practice) I settled down. Just standing there, my heart slowed down, I caught my breath, the pain subsided. Hey, I figured, I was still standing. What more do I have to worry about?

My sister, Maria, and Dad decided enough was enough. Time to go home. So I gradually and gently glided down to the bottom without a lot of exertion. I felt fine again. The pain was gone and my heart was back to its previous level of pounding in my ears. But this time, not so loud and hard that I was worried about it. I even carried my nephew out to the car with him over one shoulder and our skis and poles over the other. Then I drove home.

Maria insisted that I meet with a colleague of hers in Albany. A heart specialist. So I accepted her invitation to make an appointment for me. She did so and by noon the next day, I had an appointment for Tuesday, February 1.

Well, as you'll come to learn more about, I had created an organization called Rock2Rebuild a few weeks earlier in response to the horrible tragedy of the tsunami in south Asia. Hundreds of thousands of people were dead and tens of thousands of children were orphaned, homeless and in serious jeopardy from starvation, disease and predation. I was a man on a mission. A few days after the disaster, I recruited a colleague of mine in the music business, Jeff Mirel, to rally local music lovers to employ what we knew – music - in aid of these kids. We had a major concert event planned at Albany's historic Palace Theatre for February 11, just ten days away. I had a long list of things "To Do".

I skipped the appointment my sister had made special arrangements for me to get. I skipped it. Let me repeat that. I had what I thought was a heart attack on Sunday and on Tuesday I skipped a doctors appointment that my sister made special arrangements for me to get. I know, I know: Stupid! What did I tell you?

I emphasize this because I think we can all relate to this just a little bit. O.K. Maybe not to this extremely stupid extent, but be honest, how many times have you made a decision that was contrary to your health and well-being because you were busy with things on your TO DO list!?

My sister was fuming.

Maria: "I've made another appointment for you with the heart doctor. If you miss that appointment, I'll kill you myself!"

On February 3rd, I was at Dr. Lou Papandrea's office in Albany. He ran tests. EKG, EEG, Echo, blah, blah, blah. I didn't go to medical school. He ran tests. Dr. P tells me that from the outside, I appear to be a "normal", healthy, fit, 40-year-old male (there was that 40 thing again!). BUT, clearly, the symptoms I was describing were anything but "normal". He explained that the only way to be sure that my heart wasn't suffering from a blockage of some sort was to go into my arteries and take a look.

I said that I thought that made sense. A little scary but sensible. He explained he'd like to schedule a procedure in which he would explore the arteries supplying blood to the muscles of my heart and if necessary install devices designed to hold them open. The procedure is called a cardiac catheterization and these devices are called stents. They're installed by the thousands every day across North America.

"Well, I've got a big concert coming up in 8 days, is there any way we could do this stent thing after that?" I asked.

"George," he looked at me with mild disgust (the way I remember the school librarian looking over her bifocals at me when I'd disrupted things. You don't recall that look? O.K. I guess that was just me.). "I'd do this procedure TODAY if I could get you into the O.R. today!"

I accepted his advice, had my blood drawn in the lab for the anesthesiologist's purposes and met with the nurse to go over the instructions for taking blood thinners, etc. for the next morning's 7 AM procedure.

About two hours later (honestly, it could have been five minutes, it could have been half a day, time was a bit distorted at this point) my cell phone beeped to let me know that my current concert-planning phone-call was being interrupted by another incoming call. I was directly in front of the Albany Medical Center Hospital. I recognized the phone number as that of my new cardiologist and took the call.

"George, it's Lou…Papandrea."

"I've got good news and some concerns. Your heart's fine. What I can't figure out is why – according to your blood tests – you have about 20% of the effective blood that you should have. In fact, usually the people with these kinds of numbers I've seen have been unconscious."

"Ooooh Kaaay?"

"You need to get to a hospital and get some transfusions and we need to figure out what's causing these numbers. We need to find you a hematologist."

"Is this something I have to do today or can I do this next week? After the concert?"

"George," Lou punctuated, the frustration in his voice more than evident, "If you're alive in a week, you can get the transfusions in a week."

"Gotcha! I'm on my way home. I gotta get my kids squared away and I'll get right on it. Transfusions and a hematologist! Thank you Doctor!"

iCanSir!

I called my dad. "Do we know any hematologists?"...

At about 3 PM that same day, I was admitted through the emergency department to the Albany Medical Center Hospital about 8 miles from my kids and my home. My body had been living on borrowed time. The banker had come calling to collect.

No wonder my heart and lungs had become used to screaming for oxygen, my organs were like the littlest kids in a family of ten growing boys around the dining table, fighting for every scrap of nourishment. Literally!

From that moment, my blood was tested daily. Sometimes multiple times in a day. I kept track of my blood counts and other things on whatever scrap paper was handy. This was my first entry.

Thursday, 3 February, 2005
Hemoglobin 4.4
Hematocrit 12
WBC 2.2
Platelets 30[2]

Diagnosis: Pancytopenia
Cause: Unknown
Plan: Transfuse, examine cells
Journal Entry that day: Journal Entry? Are you kidding me? I could barely keep my eyes open. Do you honestly think I was about to start a journal? ;-) Actually, I recognized early on that a journal would be a really good idea but I just wasn't ready that first day. I would start my daily log the next day.

---

[2] For the curious: "Normal" values for these might be: Hemoglobin – 12-15, Hematocrit around 40, WBC – 3-5000, Platelets - 70

Now during this whole thing Rock2Rebuild[3] was well under way in planning the Palace concert. I had also just completed the recording, mixing and packaging of my record label's first compilation CD[4]. I was managing the growth of my law practice, my consulting firm, Leadership Motivation, LLC. and trying to complete a second book about goal setting. All this craziness on top of raising my two great kids, which is <u>really</u> my full time career! I was working long, hard hours and I was tapped out! I was exhausted constantly. By the time I got to the hospital it was all I could do to stay awake at 3 o'clock in the afternoon.

After just 2 transfusions[5], however, I felt like superman! Contrasted to just days before, I was operating on at least 4 cylinders and I felt wonderful. They told me I still had no immune system so I had to be careful about walking around the hospital too much. So, I waited until the wee hours when it was quiet and I could make tracks. I didn't want to be like the character "Papillion" and have the four walls of my room make me crazy! I was determined to stay as active as possible and get out and around whenever I could.

At midnight or so, I'd walk around the hospital. It's absolutely huge. The whole building has five or six wings to it so a person could walk for a week and not see the whole thing. Each time I'd walk, I'd explore a bit farther and then return to my room. Each time returning under the "Cancer and Blood Disorders Center" sign that hung from the ceiling in the hallway outside my room. There was another sign

---

[3] Take a look: www.rock2rebuild.org.

[4] Decaffeinated is a project of which I am very proud. A group of incredibly talented local musicians (singer, songwriters) and I got together and made a nice collection of tunes inspired by the "coffee house" environment. This wonderful and thoroughly listenable collection is available at www.yodelingloonrecords.com.

[5] 2 of the 8 transfusions that I was to receive during my month-long stay in the Bone Marrow Transplant Unit (BMTU as I came to know it).

nearby which also read "BMTU", Bone Marrow Transplant Unit. This sign designated the five or six private rooms along their own little hallway, each with special equipment to accommodate the extra precautions necessary for someone whose immune systems were in rough shape (like mine).

Just as my vital signs had been figuratively everywhere the week before, these material signs were literally everywhere. Just as my symptoms had been in my face for over a year, these signs were right in front of me! But I still didn't get it.

Friday, 4 February, 2005
Diagnosis: One of a family of 100 or so lympho-proliferative blood disorders
Plan: Continue transfusions, establish diagnosis
Cause: Unknown

Quote of the day:

"Lymphoproliferatives respond nicely to treatment."

Dr. Peter Burkart

Journal Entry:

I gratefully accept this blood as a gift from the universe and send energy of gratitude to those people who brought this new life to me.[6] I understand that just as surely as my body can – for whatever reason, "willy nilly" – shut

---

[6] I kept a list of people who I'd imagined had donated their blood for me. People in the rock world like David Lee Roth, Mick Jagger, Keith Richards, Neil Peart, Pete Townsend, Steven Tyler, Joe Perry...you get the picture. It was a real who's who of rock!

down the production of important cells, it can with equally apparent caprice restart that production. I intend for my marrow right here, right now to produce those healthy cells.

I am on a mission to help my loved ones and as many other people as possible to morally & ethically accomplish the great things we're meant to.

I am creating balance in my life! I am producing health, strength and power! I take care, take risks and enjoy!

I live with Vigor!

For three days and three nights I walked underneath those signs and not once had it dawned upon me that I had anything other than a case of "tired blood". Whatever the hell that meant. No one had ever said "tired blood" to me or anything like that, I just figured since I was so tired all the time and everything seemed to be pointing to my blood, it sort of made sense. It's a damn good thing I didn't go to medical school after all. "A couple of transfusions and I would be fine", I told myself under my still labored breath. I honestly thought that the only reason they put me in the BMTU (Bone Marrow Transplant Unit) was because that's where my old family friend and now hematologist, Dr. Peter Burkart, usually happened to be as a faculty member and attending physician. Heck, until they told me about my compromised immune system, I thought I had a private room because they'd rolled out the red carpet for Dr. Kansas' kid! Even then, I just thought that there happened to be a room available there in what I knew to be a very busy hospital.

I honestly figured that after a quick oil change, I'd be back out on the road!

iCanSir!

Chapter Three
A side-bar on humor.[7]

It was Friday. I had only been in the hospital one night at this point. Although I'd been there less than 24 hours, I'd been stuck with a needle at least a dozen times already. Intravenous tubes for nutrition, hydration and transfusion had all been hooked up. I was wondering when they were going to come in and change my transmission fluid!

At this point, you may recall, we knew that I was dealing with some type of lympho-proliforative disorder. That's something that had permeated my lymph system and disrupted the normal operation of my blood supply. The hows and whys, we didn't yet know. I mentioned that there are a hundred (give or take) potential such disorders. The next step was to narrow it down. Doctors are an amazing bunch of scientists. As a scientist myself (you didn't know I was a double-major in college, did you?[8]) I was fascinated by the step-by-step approach my team took to identify what was making me so sick. It also helped me to prepare as I understood what each step was designed to do. I think it's a good thing to have a grip on the plan. It helps the patient to be involved and understand what's going on.

So they'd done a bunch of blood tests. They'd done blood counts and cell analysis from which they'd determined that my red blood cells

---

[7]A "side-bar" is a term of the legal arts describing when a lawyer or lawyers are called to or asked to approach the judge for a brief conference out of hearing of the jury and court stenographer. The discussion is off the record and therefore physically accomplished on the side of the judges bench. Thus, it is called a "side-bar". My Editor, Denny, tells me that this is also a common expression used by authors to describe this type of story. I never knew that.

[8]I graduated from Hartwick College with two majors, one in Business/ Entrepreneurship and one in Ecology/Natural History. The science part of it was a holdover from my first year in college as a pre-med student.

were misshapen and not fully developed. They'd determined that I had way too many white blood cells that were crowding out my red ones. Red blood cells are responsible for carrying oxygen through your body. That explains my not being able to get enough air. When you heart doesn't get enough oxygen, it pumps faster. That explains the heart pounding.

Next, we had to determine what was causing all of this disruption. Since it was a blood issue, and blood is created in the bone marrow, the bone marrow was our next stop. Now, this was something I didn't know. Your bone marrow does most of its blood production in the pelvis, the hands and the spine. I had always thought it was in your arm and leg bones but apparently this is no longer thought to be true. Anyhow, the pelvis was our next stop. Oh, lucky me.

Did I mention that Albany Medical Center is a teaching hospital? It happens also to be where both my father and my sister graduated from medical school. Well, being a guest in a teaching hospital means that if it's o.k. with you, they'll march a whole troupe of medical students, interns and residents through your room (and your body) so that they can learn from your experience too. I was all for this. Knowing how important it is for doctors of the next generation to have a sense of what the patient is going through and how that patient's attitude can make all the difference, I figured "I'm gonna teach these people something!"

So on Friday morning Dr. B came in with a half dozen medical students. I'm my usual gregarious self and greeted them all with a bright "Good morning!" I'm pretty sure that I was the only one who'd greeted them this way that morning because they all looked at me like I was an alien. Now they'd all heard that I was a motivational speaker and now a record producer and concert promoter so I think there might have been some undeserved mystique about my room but not being one to burst their collective bubble, I played the role of the eccentric rock'n'roller wonderfully. Earrings in place and attitude in mind, I was ready to teach these "kids" a thing or two.

Dr. B explained to me that in order to get a picture of what was going on in my pelvis (excuuuuuse me?) they needed to do what is called a bone marrow biopsy. Sounds innocuous enough. "O.K. so what's that entail?" I wondered out loud. Dr. B described the procedure in which they drill a small hole in my pelvis at the rearward portion of my hip, take a plug of bone for testing, insert a needle and draw out a sample of marrow for testing. As he described the procedure, the blood (ironically enough) drained from my face. The rock star attitude along with it.

Yikes, that sounded like it might hurt. They offered morphine to help the pain. Well, rock'n'roll attitude or not, I'm not real big on getting high unless it involves a helicopter and a pair of skis. I passed on the morphine. It wasn't machismo. It's just that I'm very sensitive to exogenous chemicals of any kind in my body. Even allergy medicine messes me up.

My sister had come to visit earlier that morning so she was still with me when Dr. B and his entourage ("my team" as I like to egocentrically call them) came in. She encouraged me to take the pain meds as she had witnessed and even performed these bone marrow biopsies before. I trusted my gut and declined again and we were ready to go.

They had me flatten my adjustable bed out, roll over onto my belly and pull my pajama pants down to expose my buttocks. I was lying there with my bare behind sticking out like, well, bare buttocks. My sister took my hand as I prepared for the local anesthetic. This would, I would soon find out, numb the skin for the incision but would do nothing for the part about drilling into my pelvic bone.

"No pictures please" I blurted to the gathering crowd around my backside. The room erupted in hysterics. Who was this crazy man and why was he joking at a time like this? Let me tell you, it's exactly times like this to break out your best material. I was scared to death. I'm not going down without getting a laugh first!

Dr. B started the procedure. The first step was the injection of the local anesthetic to numb the skin for the incision. So far, so good. Next was the incision. Only about an inch or so cut on the top of my buttock. I couldn't really feel anything then other than some pressure. Next came the insertion of the core auger into this new cut on the top of my rear. A little pressure. Core drilling. "O.K. now THIS f*#king HURTS!" This guy is putting his whole body into it. With all his weight, Dr. B is drilling into my pelvis. The sound is so very deeply disturbing. I hear this squeaking sound as the auger drills into my bone. It reminds me of when a wood screw goes into a board and starts to get really tight toward the end. I'm breathing really deep now and clutching Maria's hand and the bed side with my sweaty hands and my backside is getting a tan from the overhead light.

Man was I glad Maria was there. I'm still not sure but I may have broken her fingers in my clutch. I was squeezing her hand so tight I thought for sure I'd break something.

Dr. B inserts the needle into the cavity inside my pelvic bone and begins drawing the sample. The pain at this point is pretty much lingering from the drilling I'd just taken (literally!). I feel some clicking and some strange vibrations and then, "All set!" I hear Dr. B say. Music to my ears. Music. Music. Yeah, good time to make a music reference, maybe sell some CDs.

"O.K. now, since we're all so close, there's no excuse for everyone in this room not to go to my concert next week." Again, the room erupts in laughter as I blot the sweat from my forehead and dry my hands. As the blood returned to my sister's hand, my humor had set everyone at ease (including me). I'd shown that even when there are a lot of unknowns in the air, I could always choose my approach. I could have freaked out, taken the morphine and been high all day or I could buck up, feel the pain, enjoy the moment and make everyone laugh with my hairy butt in the air in the process. The choice was mine.

Now I'm not advocating that you decline pain medication if your pain is unbearable. I'm just saying that you can decide ahead of time what pain you're willing to bear in order to be sober enough to crack jokes. In fact, something I didn't know before this experience, scientists have proven that laughter enhances immune function and releases your body's own natural pain killers called endorphins. Without even knowing it I was applying natures oldest pain remedy. By cracking wise with my team, I was teaching them and healing me at the same time.

Of course, I've also spoken with hundreds of people who advocate taking the opportunity to use the great drugs that you might ordinarily be disinclined to use. Be it out of decorum, respect for the law, a sense of responsibility, there are people who would not partake in drugs. Given the opportunity to do so legally, however, they're all for it. Hey, more power to 'em. It just goes to show you that there are as many ways to approach something as there are people. What I advocate is that you do what you feel right about. If you want to try to tough it out to see what the pain will do to or for you, give it a try. If you don't, that's fine too. As long as you pay attention to what's happening, you can learn from it.

Often times we take life so very seriously. Sometimes that's fine. It's important when you're standing in front of a judge or an IRS auditor. The danger comes when we start to take ourselves too seriously. Life is a dangerous, exciting and funny adventure. If we don't balance our sense of humor and awe against our sense of self-importance, we'll burn out from the pressure of it. The flip side is true. When we keep things in perspective with humor and sharing with others, we can strike a healthy balance among the things we've got to handle and how we handle it.

iCanSir!

Just for giggles, take a moment to list five funny things you saw, said, heard, did or thought today?

_____

_____

_____

_____

_____

Saturday, 5 February, 2005
Journal Entry:

I have at least 2 books still in me. @ least 3 CDs still to produce. Thousands of speeches yet to give and most importantly 2 wonderful children to raise to be healthy, self actualized, interdependent people.

Golden List: (stuff I'm grateful for)

Peter & Tessa	Mom & Dad
Kids, smiles, hugs	Maria & Elaine
Health, Family	Resourcefulness
Sense of humor	Love, Wit
Creativity, Freedom	Connectivity, Support

My friends:
Stephen B., Tom C., Rick W., Jonathan P.,
Jim B., Frank F., Bruce K., T-Bone, Eric H. & Krissy G.,
Roberto, Ant, Wolff...

Chapter Four
Somebody thinks I have cancer?!

On Sunday, my family visited early. Maria brought my kids to see me. With my surgical mask on, we walked around the hospital together. We may have even stepped outside through the impressive original front entrance of the Albany Medical Center Hospital for a breath of fresh air. It's called the "crescent" entrance, by the way, because the architectural feature which characterizes it is a half circle lined with pillars, marble stairs running the entire length from one side of the semi-circle to the other. It's been overtaken by modern features such as a disabled access ramp on one side, an overhead bridge from the parking garage across the street and the enormous brick wall of the hospital's magnetic imaging center on the other. Nonetheless, it is the original entrance to one of the country's oldest teaching hospitals and when visiting, I still always like to enter the hospital through this historic doorway.

On this day, My dad and I took a walk together as well. It was a lovely walk up New Scotland Avenue that I hope I shall never forget. The road is significant for several reasons. The first is that just days ago it was where I was driving when Dr. Lou informed me of my situation. It's also special because Albany Law School, my alma mater, is directly across the street from the hospital. I walked this road many times as a younger man. This walk, on this day, was special. I remember asking my Dad if he thought I was going to die? Without really answering my question, we discussed the situation. We talked about the kids. The walk was just enough to wind me.

Then I had the day to myself. I figured it would be a good time to catch up on the sleep that my body had long been craving.

I woke up from a sound, four-hour nap and I decided to commit a few hours to quiet meditation. I started with my usual meditation techniques. First I breathe deeply. I allow my mind to go through its sort of manic reflections of the stuff on its plate. This usually lasts only a minute or so as the breathing begins to have its calming effect. I allow the various things that concern me to pop into my consciousness without getting too worried about them. I know that those things will be here for me when I come back from my mental vacation. I know that soon enough I will be beyond all of these worries as I allow my peace-inducing breathing to take over.

After the "trailer" is over, I continue as many belly breaths as I can focus on before my mind begins to wander. When I've breathed deeply a bit and I notice the first signs of my mind wandering, I begin to think about what "nothing" looks like. I imagine my eyes watching a movie screen set up in the front of my head. I imagine what "nothing" being projected onto that screen would look like. If you've never done it, it's easier than you might imagine. It just takes a little practice.

I usually do this for as long as I need to really settle myself down. Sometimes just a minute or two will get me right back into a nice state for productivity or focus or conversation or writing or sex or whatever I am shifting gears to do.

On this day, I put in a good couple hours or so of this. "Nothing, nothing, nothing." Two hours of solid breathing. Inhaling peace and calm and serenity and exhaling agitation and stress and anxiety. In and out. In and out. Like the wonderful rhythm of the ocean or a gentle mountain breeze or lovers intertwined. Nice and easy and calm. Nothing gets me in the zone like taking the time to do this. It's the best investment I can make in myself. On this day, I was – in my mind – far from the confines of my hospital room. I had transcended – as I had done a thousand times before – the physical limitations of my now diseased body and was soaring in the ether tethered only by my love of my children and life.

Through the ether as I traveled, I was reminded of the signs in my life. Here and there ideas like altitude sickness, getting out of breath walking up the stairs, and more recent messages like "20% blood", "you should be unconscious" and "you were the one skiing with a 4 hemoglobin?" echoed in my ears. Images like the Bone Marrow Transplant Unit and the Blood Disorder and Cancer Center signs flashed like slides on the screen in my head. Punctuating the peace and calm were profound and not-so-subtle hints that things were not well within my physical body.

Then, after what felt like many relaxing hours of this wonderful transcendence, through the mist of "nothingness" I had conjured, the universe sent me a message. It hit me. It hit me like the proverbial "ton of bricks". My eyes snapped open and I froze. I think if the nurses had come into my room at that moment, they would have seen the iconic light bulb illuminated and suspended above my head.

"Somebody thinks I have cancer?!"

I may even have said it out loud. I'm sure I must have at least whispered it to myself.

Not really knowing what else to do at that point, I thought on it and thought on it. I got quiet again and just breathed. I let myself open to the sounds of the universe. I listened for the humming, felt for the vibration, made myself open to the inspiration.

After I had meditated on my situation, I sat there and let it sink in. I came to understand that it was me this time who faced a challenge. At that moment, I didn't know exactly what the challenge was going to be called, but I knew a challenge lay ahead of me.

I knew it was me, this time, whom I needed to coach. After over ten years of coaching people in how to perform at higher levels in all areas of their lives, in a matter of a few short hours, I had become my own client. It wasn't a stranger who had come to me with a life challenge to figure out. It was me.

As I mentioned in Chapter 1 - "Always", just a few years before, my mother had been diagnosed, was treated for and succumbed to a very aggressive form of cancer. In a few short months she found out, fought hard and died. It was almost 5 months from the date of her diagnosis to her death. As it was for my mother, of course, it was a profound experience for my whole family and me. I'd read that it's normal for survivors and family members of beloved cancer patients to experience a sort of "diagnostic panic" when they sense something's wrong for years after the initial cancer experience.

You have a bout of gas and you think, "I have colon cancer!" Or you get a headache and right away it's a tumor. You have a stitch in your side and you think "My God, it's my pancreas!" On the one hand it's ridiculous. I mean, four years ago, I didn't even know where the hell my pancreas was. On the other hand, it happens to a lot of people. Something is off, you think "it's cancer". The ironic thing is that often times when people are diagnosed with advanced cancer, it turns out that they had ignored symptoms because they didn't want to be hypochondriacs.

As soon as I put these signs together and figured out that I might have cancer, the first thing I thought was that it was "Mom's cancer". It made sense to me, given my frame of mind and the goings-on of the past several months (exhaustion, discomfort, etc.).

It may seem a little crazy, perhaps, that I didn't get scared. I didn't panic.

Because I had invested the previous ten years or so of my life to understanding what it took to know peace and had never been afraid to really take an honest look inside, I knew that I had to come to terms with it. I had read enough books and worked with enough people to know that the longer I wasted my time fussing over what to worry about, the longer I'd be postponing my own recovery. I dedicated the next few hours to meditating on my life and how it might end - and how soon!

Into the evening, I continued my peaceful meditation. In and out. Deep, deep breaths. In with the peace and calm and healing energy and out with the toxic and stress and negative energy. I was amazed at my ability to remain focused on my inner self for such a long period of time. Of all the years I had been meditating, I had never focused my peace and breathing for such an extended effort. The results were well worth it.

I decided that I had three potentialities to accept.

One was that the worst-case scenario was a terminal diagnosis in which case I may expire in six months just as my mother had done a few years earlier. A second was that I was absolutely fine. The third was that I was seriously ill, I had cancer of some kind, and that I would survive but with a tough road ahead of me.

I decided that if I could come to grips with each of those scenarios - and truly accept them, and fast - I could accomplish anything. I figured the sooner I could free myself from denial and accept these possibilities, the sooner I could be honest with myself about a plan.

I set to meditating on each of these new potentialities. I focused on understanding this new set of possibilities. I sought to embrace my new paradigm.

I knew that the Jumper Cables for the Soul® program I had taught to thousands of people over the years would help. I didn't exactly know how, but I knew it would. I figured, why the hell had I been investing so much time and energy into it if it wouldn't help me NOW?

So, I took myself through my own program. The one I've been teaching and working at and fine-tuning for over a decade. The same program essentially that you're going through in this book. I gave myself my own Jumper Cables for the Soul® speech. I applied it to myself. I heard my words from a new perspective (as a client this time).

I'm going to take you through the extremely condensed version of this program in this chapter. These first steps are the foundation upon which I built my recover and upon which you can build yours. I came to some important observations after completing this while in the hospital and it will help you understand why I was able to do that once you've done it at least once. The whole process will take you less than 10 minutes.[9]

I recalled the many times I'd asked my audiences to take one minute to write all of the things they would seek to accomplish if they absolutely knew that failure was not possible. What would they reach for if they knew their success was guaranteed? I call this our Lottery List. What would you do if money was no obstacle? We've all gone through these scenarios, haven't we? What would you do if you knew you'd earn what you needed to earn and learn what you needed to learn?

Right now, take one minute to write as many items as you can think of, that you would seek to see, be, do or have in your lifetime as though you absolutely could not fail. As though your success was guaranteed. Remember, it doesn't have to be perfect. You can edit this list later as I'll ask you to do many times over the next several weeks.[10] Just put 60 seconds on the clock, put your pencil to paper and start writing. Go!

_____

_____

---

[9] In fact, the trademark for the original program I taught ten years ago was *Eight minutes to change your life!*

[10] Once you've accomplished this list and the lists following it, I'll ask you to repeat this exercise everyday for a week, every week for a month and every month for the rest of your life.

_____

_____

_____

_____

Excellent! Well done!

Now, take another minute to write all of those things you would seek to see, be, do or have over the next <u>three years</u> as though your success was guaranteed. This time, though, there's a catch. This time, I'm asking you to write all of those wonderful things you'd seek to see, be, do or have AND you knew today that at the end of those three years you would be struck by a bus and killed (yikes!). I call this one the City Bus List.

_____

_____

_____

_____

_____

_____

Excellent again! Well done! I've found that this one gets us to sharpen our pencils. If you're like most people, the priorities may have changed a bit. In my audience workshops I ask folks to show hands to let me know who had priorities change from the first list to the second. For a lot of people the second list is simply shorter. That's o.k. too. There are no wrong answers. That's why I call these simply lists, not tests! See? Easy!

When my mom was ill, there came a point in her therapy when she decided to leave the hospital. It was right before Christmas and she came to a decision to go home, stop her treatment, invest whatever time she had left to being with her family in her home and enjoy the holidays as best she could. We knew what she wanted and to the extent that we had any right to, we got our minds around it and "gave her permission" to make that decision.

The day Mom was ready to go home, I waited with her in her hospital room while my dad finalized the discharge papers. I'll cherish those moments we invested together that day at St. Peter's Hospital in Albany. My mom sat on the edge of her bed and she looked at me and said words that echo in my head.

She said "George, don't put things off!"

To this day, when I find myself hesitating to do something I know to be the right thing to do, I hear her words. They inspire me to take action. For years I wasn't sure exactly why she told me this other than to inspire me. Then one day during a seminar it hit me. I used to ask my audiences to write all of the things they'd hope to accomplish over the <u>next</u> 90 days. This was very effective for years. Then one day, after this incident, I realized how much more powerful it would be if we added the little twinge of potential regret. By putting ourselves at the edge of the bed <u>right now</u>, and asking ourselves to <u>look back</u> 90 days instead of forward, we sharpen the pencil even more!

Now - quickly - answer this question. Put yourself sitting on the edge of your bed, believing your time on this earth was rapidly drawing to a close (at this point in my experience it wasn't that hard to do) what would you look back on the <u>past</u> 90 days and wish you had done?

Write all of those things here:

_____
_____
_____
_____
_____
_____

Now, if you're like 99% of the people in my audiences, I'll wager that on this list, you had items that fit one of three categories: 1) Doing something with another person. 2) Saying something to another person. Or 3) Doing something you consider crazy (like jumping out of an airplane)![11]

As I sat there on my bed recalling the many talks my Mother and I had during her final weeks and how they had inspired me, I completed this exercise for the umteenth time. The answers came out of me as naturally as my own name.

The reality of this was that I realized that I had made some outstanding choices in my life. I may not have been rich as some people may measure it. I may not have done everything right as a dad and as a former husband, as a son, a brother, or even boyfriend to the "ex"es since my marriage failed 10 years ago. But as a dad, my most important role, I had done the right thing more often than not. I took stock of my life. On the whole, I was pleased with what I saw. Not every little detail, of course, but overall, I was pleased.

If, while reading this, you can't say that now, don't worry. By the time you you're finished with this book, you'll be on the way to saying so.

---

[11] About five weeks later, upon leaving the hospital and then driving my car for the first time in weeks, the very first song I heard while driving was Tim McGraw's "Live like you were dying!" To this day, it's one of my favorite songs. A kind of anthem for me. The lyrics are right on track. The song tells the story of a man who learns the power of leading his life as though he was dying. If you don't own it, I encourage you to buy it and listen to it. As an independent record producer who has worked with many talented musicians, I feel strongly about paying for the music I enjoy. So don't bootleg, please buy it! Whatever riches come to Tim McGraw for making such a song, he's earned every cent of it!

The reality was that when I asked these questions in what I thought was the context of my imminent death, the answers were not haunting and remorseful but rather they were liberating and truly inspired. I have to say that this was one of the top six most profound moments of my life so far.[12]

I came to the conclusion that if I was going to expire in 6 months I could do so in peace, knowing that - although I really, really, really, really, really, really didn't want to - I could, because I had set an outstanding example for my children.

This freed me to make an amazing decision.

My work was not yet finished. I simply couldn't quit yet. Understand that I didn't say to myself, "I'm not going to die" or anything quite that dramatic. How could I know that? How can any of us know? I did say, however, that I was not done yet. I could know that!

I had work yet to do. I didn't know how long I had to do it but I knew I had it to do. Whatever remaining time I had - one day, one month, one year - didn't matter. The time I did have, would be committed to doing what I'd been doing. Teaching my kids, helping people, changing the world.

In fact, my personal mission statement had been for years "to enthusiastically guide my children, my loved ones and as many other people as possible to morally and ethically accomplish the great things they're meant to."

---

[12] I have to say that the other five are probably in chronological order 1) the birth of my son, 2) the birth of my daughter, 3) the day I became sole custodial parent of my kids, 4) the last conversation I had with my Mom and 5) the moment immediately before finishing my first marathon race just 23 months after my diagnosis.

iCanSir!

I was determined to continue this "work" with every breath I had left. Be it 1 or 1 billion breaths. I had to create a mindset to give my body the best chance to heal so that I could teach my children some more for as long as I could. I had to give myself the best chance of healing so I could continue this work. Getting my mind in the right frame of mind was my first priority. After a long, deep look into the recesses of my mind through meditation, the result was the most incredible, powerful, balanced, certain peace I'd ever experienced. That's the peace I want you to be able to find too. I want the world to know it. I think that's my mission here. I reach for and teach that incredible, overwhelming, calming and reassuring peace. If that kind of certainty is what you think you crave, read on. If not, read on anyway. You'll learn something. I promise.

Here's what I wrote in my makeshift journal at the end of all this pondering.

Journal Entry:

I can stand up - and through each of my cells figuratively stand up - and say NO you do not belong here. Cancer cells you are disrupting the natural order of things. I am in charge here. You are here uninvited. I stare you down with certainty. I show no fear because I feel none. I am right. I express no fear, no hesitancy because I experience none. These healthy and unhealthy cells are within my dominion. I will evict the unhealthy ones. You will not win because it is simply not the order of things. It is the order of things for me to know health and you are put on notice. I have the God energy on my side and you will perish. I will prevail because my will prevails. Bottom line – I am better than you. You may be strong, but I am resourceful. You may be clever, but I am intelligent. You may be wily, but I am agile. You may

51

be one tough motherf*#ker but I am the baddest motherf*#ker any cancer cell has ever seen. I'll beat you. You can go quietly or you can go with a fight but GO... YOU... WILL!

Yeah, there may be a bit of denial in there. Maybe. But it's pretty powerful stuff for a start. For me, it created a very clear image. Wouldn't it be great if everyone receiving a diagnosis that isn't so good could feel this way going into it? It is possible. You see, I'm not any different than you or anyone. I just prepared myself a little unconventionally. You can too.

Doctors are amazing. The drugs are amazing. The nurses are amazing! But you know what? So is my body. So is yours. So are all of ours! Our minds are even more amazing than that! I believe that my decision to be certain in at least the idea that no matter how much time I had I knew what I was going to do with it had something to do with my impressive recovery.

In fact, there exist tons and tons of good science in the field of healing and in the area of quantum physics that support the concept that just the idea of my being well, helped to make me well. More on this later.

The end to this long chapter, my friend, is this...

The next day Maria came to visit. She brought a donut and a decaffeinated cup of coffee for me and we sat and talked. She said to me, "Why is this happening to you, George?"

Without a moment's hesitation I answered her. "Because I can handle it, Maria" was my reply with an almost stoic certainty.

iCanSir!

"Because I can handle it." I echoed.

Although you may not be mindful of it right now, you can handle it too! You wouldn't be reading this book right now if that weren't true.

Chapter Five
A diagnosis by any other name...

I sincerely believe, deep, deep in my bones, that what befalls us, befalls each of us for our own reasons. Of course, along with this belief – in order to maintain our sanity – must necessarily come the realization that it may not ever make absolute sense to us during our physical lifetime. In fact, it often doesn't.

It certainly seems impossible to explain why horrible things happen to children, for instance. In the struggle to understand it, however, we may yet get a glimpse of that magical stuff of the universe. That of which we are truly made.

Put another way, the key isn't in the understanding, it's in the trying to get it. It's not in the goal, it's in the pursuit of the dream.

Aristotle is quoted as having said that "the unexamined life is one not worth living." In my experience, it is certainly true that the human condition is improved when it is examined. When approached with mindfulness, that condition is one of what I call "emotional archaeology". Digging and sweeping. Digging and sweeping. In an intermittent and never ending search to uncover the origins of the ideas that drive our own behavior, our personal existence, our unique truth.

I made some observations during my digging and sweeping that may guide you in yours. This digging and sweeping really opened my eyes to what was going on inside my body. The approach I took to my treatment was a direct result of these discoveries or observations. I'm sure this made a difference. I believe that the certainty I was able to garner as a direct result of all of this digging and sweeping is what made it possible for me to survive. I'm certain that it helped. It certainly didn't hurt! Everyone who really knows me and who really knows what I went through and how I have lived my life certainly believes that it did. Hell, my doctors even said my attitude had a lot to do with my recovery. I guess it's true then.

I mentioned earlier that I knew that I had to come to grips with some profound realities. I knew I had to do it but I didn't know how. Through the course of that digging and sweeping, I came across these "hows". You are benefiting from my experience by skipping directly to those hows by applying what I've written here directly into your life. Know that it works. Is it curing your cancer? I truly wish I knew. Do I hope it helps you do this? Of course. I don't want anyone suffering from any member of this family of diseases any longer than is absolutely necessary for you to learn what it is the universe intends for you to learn.

So, what WILL it do? It will help you to weather the suffering you'll endure in your life. It will help you discover and maintain your inner certainty. It will help you help your family and loved ones deal with what you're dealing with too.

Yes, I know I said "necessary" up there about the suffering. It might not be a popular idea but some amount of suffering is necessary for us to learn what we need to learn. I've done some of mine and I'm certain I'll do more. You'll do yours. We all do our own suffering at one point or another.

It comes in varying degrees and at different times. It comes without warning, without preparation, without instructions. Now, however, you'll be armed with the benefit of my experience! You'll go in stronger, you'll deal with it smarter, you'll come out better! I know this takes courage. I won't play down how difficult it is to do the digging and sweeping. It's not only important, though, it's worth it! The joy and balance and peace and inspiration and understanding that come from this courageous and sometimes painful endeavor can be amazing. It can not only change your life but also multiply the impact you have on others. Again, I've been there. I know you may be thinking that this is just too big right now. I know it's scary. I really do. Keep going. Whatever it takes. Reach down into your soul and find the strength. If it's not there, keep going anyway. All the answers may not be at your fingertips right now. You can trust me when I say that right now, you don't need all the answers. Tomorrow may bring more answers: it may not. The answers, the information will come as you need it. You may think you need more right now. And you may. Try to stay calm and keep breathing. You'll be able to develop a plan as you gather your information.

So, I'd gone through "the lists" as you just did in the last chapter the exercise renewed my inspiration. I'd accepted the fact that I had some kind of cancer. I'd accepted the fact that it was a possibility that I would not see my 41st birthday just 6 months away. I'd accepted the fact that I'd need to make the absolute most of these days, many of which I'd likely invest[13] in the hospital, regardless of whatever outcome awaited me. Now, in the very short term, I would await the "official" diagnosis with as much patience and balance as possible - and try not to revert to a panic in the meantime.

On Monday, the day after I'd done all of this meditation and journaling, my dad and I had been hanging out talking about my thoughts from the night before. We discussed mom and the ideas I had come up with and what he thought about it. My dad told me that because of my symptoms and where I'd ended up in the hospital (BMTU), he had a sense of what was going on. Later on I found out Maria had felt the same thing. This, apparently, is what inspired her inquiry as to why it was happening to me. Both my dad and Maria had figured out the whole cancer connection days before I had. What I had to meditate to connect, they had connected almost immediately.

---

[13] A long time ago I learned the power of our vocabulary and its effect on our actions and outcomes. I stopped using the word "spent" when referring to my time and my life. I've found that I prefer investing my time rather than spending it. When you go to the store to spend your money, are you happier afterwards? When you invest in an enterprise that succeeds and it pays you dividends, doesn't that feel better?

iCanSir!

Dr. Burkart came into my room. This time he had the lab results from the bone marrow biopsy. "Well George we've identified what it is that's been causing the problem with your blood," he started. "When we did the biopsy we weren't able to come up with a sample to test. It's what's called a 'dry tap'. With the bone marrow gone, there's not a whole lot there to test. But we've had a good look at your cells, and we've all taken a look at the slides. The combination of symptoms, combined with your enlarged spleen and the dry tap points to a disease called Hairy cell leukemia..."

Diagnosis: Leukemic Reticular-endotheliosis
                    (Hairy Cell Leukemia)
Plan: Chemotherapy (7 day, 24 hour infusion of 49 milligrams of Leukostatin/Cladribine)
Comments to Doctor Burkart:

"I never thought I'd be relieved to hear I have Leukemia"

Journal Entry:

It's not "I'm not going to die" or "this isn't going to kill me."

It's "I'm alive, I'm well, I am strong, I am resourceful. I can handle anything."

It's called Hairy Cell Leukemia because under a microscope the tiny mutated white blood cells that end up overpopulating the blood and marrow (crowding out and choking off the production of healthy blood) look like tiny fuzzy tennis balls. It seems funny to me - and it seemed funny to me then - that I would end up with a disease that manifests itself in the form of blood cells masquerading as hairy

balls? I don't know, maybe it's just me and my sick sense of humor.[14]
Perhaps even more important than thinking this is funny, is
understanding that by finding humor in it, by finding the 'silly' in it, I
was able to accept it. By accepting it, I was able to begin the process
of influencing my experience actively.

---

[14] There's actually another funny story about this ironic play on words involving
an old friend, a speakerphone and a nurse. See the journal entries for Day 4 of the
workbook portion of this book. Page 134.

Chapter Six
No matter what…

Profound realization Number 1: I have cancer in my body. Like it or not, ready or not, I have cancer in my body. BUT, that's the only place it is.

Cancer. It's THE bad news. There is, however, definitely some good news, and I will share that with you in a few pages. It's best for you to get your head around the bad part first. The good news will mean more to you if you do. Unfortunately, there's no two ways about this realization. It sucks. It sucks to have cancer. Diagnosis sucks. Treatment sucks. Nausea, dizziness, diarrhea, it all sucks. Go ahead and say it out loud, it's o.k. Cancer sucks! It's really o.k. I'm giving you permission. Cancer sucks moose poop! Cancer _____ (fill in your own expletive here).

You've got to come to grips with this as quickly as possible. This chapter will help by helping you to understand the limitations of the diagnosis. It will also help if you can try not to beat yourself up for wanting to freak out in the first place. That part, at least, is a natural response to the stress of the news. But we can do better than that!

Psychologists tell us that it's "normal" to go through various stages before we accept this. It's "normal" to deny that you have anything wrong. It's "normal" to be angry. It's "normal" to negotiate with God over the outcome of your treatment. It's "normal" to get depressed.

Well, I've never been a big fan of "normal".[15] Don't misunderstand me. I'm a real believer in the good work of psychologists and believe that this information is very valuable in helping us understand the human condition. In fact, this book is meant to be but another set of

---

[15] Because we lived a little differently and my kids always expressed themselves creatively, they would be subject to the occasional jibe about being "weird". We had a standard family response to this. "Thanks, what's it like to be normal?"

observations to help us do that. It's just that despite the fact that there are lots and lots of people who have to deal with this disease, there's really nothing "normal" about being told you have cancer!

According to the dictionary, the definition of "normal" in its most common context is "conformity to a regular pattern". Now, cancer of some sort will affect one in three people. Meaning that out of every three people, one of them will either experience cancer personally or know someone closely who will experience it personally. Statistically, I'll concede that these numbers may reveal a "regular" pattern. To each of us as individuals, however, cancer's effects are not an everyday occurrence. Cancer's effects do NOT conform to our regular patterns as individuals.

So, I say…

To hell with normal.

Again, get your arms and mind around the idea that you have cancer. Now, I'm talking about accepting the <u>diagnosis</u>. I am NOT talking about accepting the whole package of what you "think" cancer is "supposed" to mean. For example: Accepting that the doctors just told you that you have cancer makes sense BUT you don't have to accept a death sentence. This will help.

A diagnosis is merely a professional observation of the condition of your physical body at a given moment in time.

Let's be honest, I had to ask myself whether I might die. Honestly, to be true to myself, I even had to answer that I might. Could I have died? Yes, of course. Was I prepared for it? To the extent that one can be, yes. "Could you die?" Yes. We're all going to die someday. Physically, at least. BUT, one could JUST AS EASILY ask the

iCanSir!

question, "Could I live?" and the answer to that question would, of course, also be "Yes, I could live!" Of course.

So let's learn to ask the right questions, shall we? Instead of "could I die?" Let's learn to ask, "Could I live?" And while we're at it, let's learn to answer, "Yes, I can live!"

When you're car shopping, you don't go looking for a lemon, do you? I mean, taken to the absurd to prove the point, imagine the look on his/her face if you asked a car salesperson "Does it stall with predictability? Will it fail to start when I need it to? Will it leak oil reliably?" Crazy right? So why would we ask such crazy questions when our lives are on the line? If we were in our right mind, we wouldn't. So, let's get into our right mind.

We're getting closer to the good news. Right now, I'm just trying to get you to accept the diagnosis and nothing more or less. Accept it for what it is. A diagnosis is just an observation about the condition of your body at a particular point in time. That's all it is. Scientifically, that's all it is.

Say it out loud.

"My diagnosis is just an observation about the condition of my body at this point in time."

In fact, technically speaking, the diagnosis is just an observation about the condition of your body in the past. Up until the time of your examination or when the tests were performed. Even if you were just examined five minutes ago, the diagnosis is still just an assessment of what the condition of your body <u>was</u>, NOT what it <u>can be</u>!

There is, however, a huge difference between the condition of your <u>body</u>, and the condition of your <u>mind</u>. Huge difference. It is possible for your body to be in one condition and your mind to be in another.

It is possible for you to experience pain and at the same time be mindful of positive emotions.

If this doesn't make sense to you, let me ask you; Have you ever laughed so hard your belly hurt? Have you ever had an orgasm and a back or leg muscle spasm/cramp at the same time? See what I mean?

O.K. you've been patient and taken the bad news like a real trooper, so here's the good news. Now say this out loud.

"No matter what happens to my body, my soul will always be cancer-free!"

The universe 'hears' our intentions without judgment about negative or positive. So to fine tune this just a tiny little bit, we can even remove the reference to cancer-free altogether.

"No matter what happens to my body, my soul will always be perfect!"

Although to a large degree the two - body and soul - are inseparable and intertwined through complex biomechanical, neuro-electrical and chemo-molecular systems that we're only beginning to understand. For the purpose of this chapter, however, I'm distinguishing your soul from your body. It's something I've done for years to help people think of their minds as something they can exert influence upon. I believe that the body also fits in this category but for now, if this is a new idea to you, it will be easier to think of the mind as a distinct field of energy from your body. It's not limited to your brain or anywhere in particular within your body.

It may be a new idea to you. It may sound perfectly fine to you. I know from my audiences that this can be a grey area for some people. You may find it hard to separate the images in your mind of your soul from your body. I believe that our bodies are living cells, which pulse with a vital energy. Our bodies (or bio-body suit as some physicists call it) are organic machines performing the various functions of life. The energy that propels them, the purpose that drives them, the thoughts, dreams and ideas that they experience, that energy - I believe - is our soul.

It is not necessary to agree with this observation in order to get the most from this book. It's just what I think is so. I could be wrong. I often am. For now, just go with it. You'll be glad you did!

So. Step one. Accept that you have cancer. It's not good, it's not bad. It's not anything but an observation about the condition of your body at this point in time. It is what it is. But also realize that the ONLY place it exists is in your body!

Now, you might not want to end this segment on that note, so consider this. No matter what the outcome of this experience, commit to the idea that you will create positive information from it.

I know from my seminars that to some of you this may seem just plain crazy. "Yeah right, I'm going to make my bleeding tumor a positive lesson in my life. Nice try Mr. Motivator guy." Believe me, I hear you on this. I've been there, remember? Please understand that I'm not saying that right this instant you have to be happy about your situation. I know I certainly wasn't. All I'm saying is that you have to trust me on the point that if you commit – or at the very least be open - to the very tiny idea that at some level you will be able to learn from this experience and that such information - at some level - will benefit your soul, you will have a much "better" cancer experience. Whatever that means to you.

You're learning many techniques that when applied in combination with your medical remedies, will strengthen your body's ability to change and to heal. As you apply these techniques, you're gaining a greater understanding of your mind's natural systems which are

iCanSir!

perfectly designed to correct problems in conjunction with your body. As you gain greater discipline over what you allow your mind to entertain, your mind plays a greater role in your healing. When you've begun the process of understanding and applying the near magical power of your mind, you'll have accomplished something grand. Your life will begin to improve in ways you wouldn't have even imagined. The people around will notice a change in you. The people around you will even appear to you to get better at being them. They'll have learned that from you!

Imagine going through this experience and finding a deeper, truer self than you knew before. Imagine going through this experience and teaching people about it in such a way as to ease their burden. Imagine being so inspired by what you learn that your legacy is magnified and leveraged exponentially as a result. Think of the people whose lives will be enhanced by your experiencing this now.

Understand that if you commit to this, your experience will not have been in vain. Your experience will have had a purpose. It's possible. For now, try to accept that too. It may help to take the sting out of it a bit. That's what I want you to take from this chapter.

> "Yes I have cancer.
> Something good will come of it and
> no matter what happens to my body,
> my soul will always be perfect."

Chapter Seven
The cancer is me.

If knowing that my soul will always be perfect is a profound realization, then this next one is a real whopper. Hold on because, at first, this one might actually be harder to swallow than accepting that you have cancer...

Profound Realization Number 2: This cancer is me. In your case, the cancer is you.

The cancer is me. Like it or not, ready or not, the cancer is me. It's not some bullet in my gut, or sliver in my foot or foreign body in my eye. These cells that are causing me problems are me. At some point in time, it took one of my own healthy cells to divide and become at least one unhealthy cell. That's what I mean by "the cancer is me".

Just like my heart, my lungs, my skin, my eyes, these little trouble makers are me too. I could have denied it all I wanted to, but it wouldn't have done me any good. You too can deny it all you want. No one would blame you. It's a big, heavy idea. In my experience, however, if you spend a lot of time in denial, you'll wish you hadn't wasted the time. I'm really hoping you'll trust me on this point especially. I had to reconcile that. You have to reconcile that too. Period. In the long run, you'll be so very glad you did.

To some, it may even seem obvious, but I've noticed that no one says it out loud. It needs to be spoken. For some reason, for most of us our minds make it tough to get. It may take a few hours to get your head around the idea. Grasping that the problems you are experiencing are coming not just from inside yourself but from your actual self is a big one to put your mind around. It's o.k. If it takes you some time to ponder this, then take the time right now.

iCanSir!

Now, keep in mind while you're doing this that I'm not saying the cancer is your fault. Fault is a word and a concept that's just loaded with judgment and you don't need to go there right now. We'll get to responsibility a bit later, but there's huge difference between responsibility and fault. Right now, just recognize that the cancer is you and that's as far as you need to go.

Come back to this when you can say and understand "The cancer is me" without feeling guilty or even going down that road. Right now, for now, you just have to be able to understand the idea. Forget about the "why" for now. Forget about the "how" for now. We'll definitely get to that. For now, just understand that "the cancer cells are tiny, tiny representations of you." Not ideal representations, admittedly. Not healthy representations, certainly, but representations nonetheless.

The cancer is me.

Ready to move on?

Let's talk about this observation's immediate implications: What could it mean? Well for starters it means that since it is you, it's really under your influence if not actual control. Like it or not, you've got the potential to have more influence over this thing than you might have believed. That, my dear friend, is good news! In fact, it's fantastic news! The idea that the cancer is you, means that you are not at the mercy of everything else in the universe. You can have an impact on your outcome! I know it may feel like you are completely dependent upon everyone else in your life right now. I know that this might make you very uncomfortable right now. Know this. Since the cancer is you, and you is your body, and your mind can influence your body, you can influence your outcome!

I know it may be a pretty huge idea to you right now. Hang on and I'll show you how I accomplished it. Of course, when I say "accomplished", I'm not necessarily talking about curing or remission. Honestly, I'd be pretty egocentric if I accepted credit for all of that. Besides, this is really not a how-to-cure-cancer kind of book as much as it is how-to-live-the-fullest-life-you-can-whether-you've-got-cancer-or-not kind of book. I was very fortunate but I also know that my focus on living well made me a better patient and one more likely to get the full benefit of all the good work my caregivers were doing. I love the Thomas Jefferson quote...

I'm a firm believer in luck.
The harder I work the more I have of it!

The harder I worked, the smarter I became. The smarter I became the more mindful I remained. The more mindful I remained, the luckier I got. The point isn't that I went into remission. I'd be writing this book even if I hadn't. I guess I just would have written it faster. The point is that I remained focused on health and determined to live true to myself throughout the process. That's what this stuff will help you do! Live true to yourself everyday. And that can only help! If you do the same thing, it will help you influence your outcome too.

Once I got my arms around the whole, "this cancer is me" thing, I knew that I needed a plan. In order to influence my outcome, I had to have a plan. In order to have a plan, I had to identify the different possibilities I might be facing.

I had to identify my worst-case scenario, accept it and formulate a plan for that contingency. I figured that if I could handle that, I'd be ready for anything. I had already, after all, accepted that I might be dead before my 41st birthday, it wasn't that much of a reach to start formulating plans in that event.

I know however, that when assessing any situation, it's important to be realistic. Nowadays in our society, when most people say "be realistic" they're saying it to bring someone down from a lofty height. But we need to be realistic in a different way. There are plenty of people in this world who will tell you that it's realistic to accept that you'll die and in a way they'll be right because eventually we all do die of something or other. I mean, how can you argue with the stats that tell us that 100% of us die of something eventually? It's like the question "why do native rain dances work?" "Because the natives don't stop dancing until it rains!" My point is that realism must also include the reality that while all of us die, all of us also are alive right this very moment. If you are reading this, you are alive. If you are alive today then two things are true: 1) You may be alive tomorrow and the next day and so on and 2) there's living to do today!

Along those lines, in reality, the potential outcomes are not only bad ones. It was just as possible that my outcome would be positive as it was that it could be negative. I also had to, therefore, identify my best case scenario, accept it and formulate a plan for that contingency as well. The funny thing was that this wasn't my first instinct. Formulating the best case scenario is usually what I'm best at. Ever the optimist, I'm usually the one identifying the silver lining in the first instance. In this case, oddly enough, the positive outcomes were the secondary prediction. Funny. It's really more important that this plan came to me at all rather than when it came.

It's also not coincidental that I thought of the worst-case scenario first. As positive a guy as I am, I'm human and I was scared. Fear has such a powerful impact. It can divert even the strongest river of love, dreams and purpose. Like a river, however, those things cannot be diverted permanently! Fortunately, I was able to wrestle the fear into submission long enough and frequently enough to be able to remain focused on the positive potential.

Finally, I had to learn from this. I had to pay attention and learn from every step of this experience. I had to keep track of my observations out of the hope that they'd be helpful. If not to me, then to someone, someday. Because I am a professional speaker, I joked with my caregivers and friends, "This is going to make a great speech someday!" I kept telling myself, "This experience is going to make a great story, book, program, etc.!" I thought of the different programs that would allow me to turn this experience into positives for the many different populations of people who were helping me. Doctors, nurses, people involved in blood donation and collection, researchers, survivors and their families, musicians. You name the demographic and I came up with a speech for them! It's one of the things that got me through it all.

As it's turned out, these notes have helped ME as much as anyone else. They've helped me keep my healthy perspective. I've returned to them many, many times and wish even that I'd returned to them even more often than I have. I pictured myself speaking to thousands of people, working with support groups, at people's bedsides. All of these images have come to pass since my recovery. I used those notes to create this book and use them nearly every day to maintain my perspective.

You may be saying to yourself "I don't need to journal my thoughts or observations or experiences, no one's going to read this stuff." That may be true. No one may ever pick up your notes or learn a thing from them. The act of writing them, however, in and of itself, will be hugely helpful.

Besides, doesn't it stroke your ego even just a little that hundreds of years after your body is dead and gone (many, many days, weeks, months, years from now!), that a great, great, great grandchild, niece or nephew or perfect stranger might pick up your journal and read it and learn about your experience and what it meant to you? C'mon be honest. Just a little?

So, you need to be realistic. The outcome could be bad. BUT, the outcome could also be good.

So prepare yourself for both contingencies.

Once I had put my head around that, I realized that either way, I had to prepare myself for my treatment. Part of that preparation was to ready my mind and body for a transformation. I had to be prepared to transform my body from one in the condition of being diseased to one in a condition of being well.

I understood that in order to change I needed to have an accurate assessment of where I was at the moment. I thought about cancer and what that might mean. I thought about what the cancer being me meant in other ways. I had always equated cancer with negativity so I thought that perhaps I had been harboring some longstanding negativity. I figured the idea that such negativity might eventually have manifested itself in my body in the form of cancer cells might not be such a stretch of the imagination.

Again, remember that these cells are me. The cancer cells in your body are you. They are our cells. They live and breathe the same air and consume the same nutrients. They are not the "enemy". They are our very selves. Somehow the process of creating cells in your body got messed up. I figured that the source of that process getting messed up in my body had to do with some kind of negativity that I had been mindful of at some point. In fact, since it was cancer and one that had manifested itself relatively slowly, the negativity I had allowed to fester was probably something I had carried for quite some time.

I had an idea in my head that it was entirely possible that over the years I had harbored enough resentment toward myself, enough self-loathing, enough disappointment with some of my choices, that I could have somehow manifested my own cancer. In a way, I thought, I could have had a hand in having created this mess for myself.

I know this might be a wild idea for some of you. I've had a lot of people suggest that I tread very lightly here. They've suggested that people might be offended at the idea that each of us could cause our own cancer. Now hold on. I'm not saying that I know for certain that each of us causes our own cancer. I'm not saying that you are responsible for giving yourself cancer. I'm not saying that, okay?

iCanSir!

What I'm saying is that we know enough about harboring negative energy to be prepared to admit to – and except some responsibility for – harboring negative energy within ourselves. I'm saying that it makes sense that if bottling up all of that negative emotion can give us an ulcer, then it's not too terrible a reach to say that it might also weaken our defenses to the point where we've made ourselves susceptible to other problems, too. Such other problems could, reasonably, include the manifestations of cancer. So don't go jumping down my throat just yet. Bear with me, this will really help you because I know there's something that you've not let go of and if I can get you to do that, you'll feel relieved and glad you did it.

So I had this idea about bottled up negativity. I thought about it. I thought about what experiences in my past might have caused me to have such negative feelings toward myself that it could have grown into this. What could have been hanging around so long that it would have an opportunity to manifest itself as cancer?

I meditated on this for a bit. It didn't take long. I didn't have to think that hard for that long. It jumped right out at me. I remembered a wrong I had perpetrated, someone I had hurt as a result of a bad decision I'd made. No one died, I hadn't committed a crime, but it did cause a lot of pain for a handful of people. It was a stupid mistake I had made in my impulsive years and it cost a small group of people a lot of anguish. I had harbored guilt about it for a long time.

I am completely unwilling to relinquish my responsibility for this. I did it. I can't deny it or pretend it didn't happen. I wish that I could deny it, deny my part in it, but that's just not how the universe operates. So without relinquishing responsibility for it, I had to come up with a way to let go of this guilt that could very well have been killing me.

Simply put, I had to forgive myself. My very life depended on it.

I meditated on accepting responsibility for what I'd done. I thought about what I had learned from it and what I could continue to learn from that experience and how to avoid it in the future. I thought about what I might do to help others avoid the same mistake. I thought about what positives could possibly come from that mistake and how I could ensure that something good did come from that. I thought about how I might make my karmic restitution.

I committed to making sure that forgiving myself wouldn't equate to just letting myself off the hook. I decided that I'd learned my lesson since having done this wrong. I decided that since that time, I had done a lot of good. I reflected on the many positives I had been responsible for since then. I thought about some of the things I had done for some of the people I had been responsible for hurting. Although, perhaps I hadn't made up for it, I felt as though I had regained some of my lost virtue.

I reflected on some of the small sacrifices I had made since then in order to see to it my children, for instance, were well taken care of. I thought about the many lessons I had since imparted on my kids to be certain (to the extent I could) that they'd not make the same mistakes I'd made. I pondered the things I could continue to do to bear this responsibility with, well, responsibility and share the lessons I had learned from all of that pain.

I felt that the sum of these things would buy me some credit. That these good deeds might help to pay down some of the "karmic debt" that might be out there as a result of my misdeeds. I hoped to forgive myself without letting myself off the hook. When I was satisfied that I had accomplished this, I moved on.

You may be asking yourself "is he going to tell us what he did or what?" No, I'm not. It's not as important as you think. If you're asking that question, you're projecting your guilt onto me in order to avoid my next question. I'm sorry, I care about you too much to let you off the hook. You've simply got to do this thinking. Remember, it just might save your life!

So here it is. What's yours? What's the guilt that has controlled you? What do you need to forgive yourself for? Look, we all have done s*#t that we regret. Anyone who tells you otherwise is trying to sell you a diet pill. So go ahead, write what you've done that you feel guilty about.

_____

_____

_____

I'm encouraging you to be honest here because keeping secrets could be what's making you ill. No one besides you ever has to see this. You can write it in code if you really don't want anyone to know. As far as I'm concerned, I won't tell anyone. In addition to being a performance coach, I'm an attorney. I've kept secrets for a living. Some of them would make your skin crawl. Trust me. No one needs to ever see anything you write in this book unless you let them.

You may be thinking "Hey, let's not get crazy here, it's not like my regrets are causing my cancer or _____"(insert your challenge here!) O.K., maybe not, but you have to admit, they sure aren't helping anything either. So, identify what you may be punishing yourself for and go about forgiving yourself.

_____

_____

_____

℟ iCanSir!

Now identify some things that you can do to alleviate some of the pain those regrets may have caused you and people you know (or people you don't know).

_____

_____

_____

Right now you may be thinking that this sounds suspiciously like one of those 12-step programs. Well I have two responses to that. The first is that when you're all done with this you can go back and count them. I guarantee you that there will be way more than 12 steps. The second is this: Yes, well, those 12-step programs have become a bit cliché because they work sometimes. Anyhow, it's still not a 12-step program so sit tight and keep reading!

I heard this guilt - this negativity - described once as "heaviness". What a burden to place upon yourself. Think about it. Can you possibly get better while carrying that extra weight on your shoulders or in your belly or in your neck muscles or wherever you carry your guilt, negativity and stress. Please accept that over the next several weeks you're going to be freeing yourself of all that extra junk.

In fact, take a moment right now to jot exactly where in your body you carry that stuff. Think about it. Do you get headaches, neck aches, stitches (cramps) in your side, back spasms, upset stomach, reflux, frequent colds, bad bowel movements? Is this starting to make a bit more sense?

Where in your body do you carry your negativity?[16]

_____

_____

_____

Now, jot some thoughts about what you might do – in addition to actively participate in this program – to process and let go of that negative energy.

_____

_____

_____

Now, jot some thoughts about what it will feel like when you've been able to do that. Mmmmm, just imagine the "lightness". Won't that feel great?

_____

_____

_____

[16] There is lots of cool information out there that correlates specific problems in the body with specific types of energy. It's fascinating to me and you may find it interesting to read up on. In many cases, this information is the result of millennia of thinking. If you're interested in checking this stuff out, a good place to start is a local holistic practitioner. I've found that these folks are tuned into a lot of the information that traditional practitioners might consider "out there" but still can be complimentary to your standard treatments. Be open with all of your caregivers. Together, you can strike a healthy balance among different approaches that works for YOU!

Do you feel a little better already? Maybe a tiny little bit?

During one of my early conversations with the intern the day before my chemotherapy was set to start, the young doctor was "sharing" his personal feeling that it was his "hope" that the chemotherapeutic agent that my doctor and I had decided on was the right one. I was furious with him. He suggested that perhaps it would take some time to be certain of the diagnosis, the treatment for which I was about to embark on a 7-day, 24-hour poison fest!

It took every ounce of self-control not to jump out of my bed and wring his neck. What a jack-ass! I was so upset that this pompous young man would place his ego before my attitude. I think his exact words were 'That's what you probably have. There's some debate about your diagnosis.' Dumb shit. Why would you say such a thing to a patient?

Well I know why he would say it. He would say it appear to more actively involved in the decisions relative to my care.He would say it to appear more intellectually involved in my care. He would say it to look smart. He would say it to check the positivity in front of him if he was uncomfortable with it. He would say if he was intellectualizing what was, for me, a very close partnership among intellect and heart.

Since that day, I've always thought that he just said that to knock me down a peg. I think, honestly, he was jealous. I think he was a little jealous that here I was at the lowest point of my life, with a smile on my face, grateful for the true blessings in my life, and he was just a miserable little turd, frustrated at being stuck in our tiny upstate New York berg. Well as far as I was concerned "tough shit". Get over it big guy. Time to cowboy up and do your job!

At the time, I refused to give him the satisfaction of engaging in a debate. I'd talk to his boss tomorrow and set him straight a little less directly right now. I said, "well, Dr. B says that's what I have and this stuff (Cladribine) will do the trick...

"we'll get the little fu@#ers!"

After I said it to him, I jotted it into my journal. It may have been crude but I can't tell you what satisfaction it gave me to show him that he and his stupid choice of vocabulary couldn't shake my confidence. So many people have told me that they've had similar experiences with their professional caregivers. Without making apologies for the occasional jack-ass, I will say that I understand that people in the health professions are worked mercilessly hard. I understand that they are not necessarily trained in the finer nuances of human interaction. Finally, I understand that they all didn't have the benefit of having been raised by my mom and dad who constantly insisted on polite and considerate behavior. Having said that, I also know that the doctors who led my team, the nurses who took care of me almost without exception, all "got it" when it came to respecting the approach I was determined to take and communicated with me accordingly.

I know many examples of extraordinary compassion and empathy in the medical profession. In my own family I'd witnessed my father, my mother, and both my sisters engage in the healing professions. At once they were all intelligent and credible and warm and compassionate. I would like to see more being taught about the importance of those skills. I remember feeling in the hospital that I'd like to deliver some programs to doctors in training to see if it would make a difference.

I will create the opportunity to make some progress in helping the health care professions understand that in each and every transaction with a patient, the way the patient will hear the information MUST be taken into account. Yes, it's harder to do it that way. Yes, it may be totally counterintuitive for those trained in the medical arts but those challenges don't make it any less important to us, the patients, and ultimately to the professionals too!

Anyhow, I'm off my soapbox now. One last thing. After having pondered the idea of having done some stupid things and having let those actions haunt me to a certain degree, I wanted to let go of it all one last time that day before I nodded off. The last note I made in my journal was to become a real mantra for me as I began my healing in earnest. I wanted to tell each and every one of my billions of cells that it was time to move on. It was time to acknowledge that this experience was something I was going to benefit from somehow. It was time to express – out loud – the thanks I felt for all the wonderful blessings I'd been able to enjoy over the years. It was time to be grateful.

It was time to let the chemicals the doctors were using do their thing. The doctors trusted these drugs to help heal me and I trusted my doctors. I'd asked the right questions, I'd educated myself and had decided to trust my team. It was time to allow my body to join that team with everything it had. It was time to let my unhealthy cells die without mourning them and move on to a new day of healing, revitalization and redemption. It was time to forgive.

"thank you – you're forgiven"

The days and weeks to follow would require every resource I had within me. Soon, in just a day or two, the anguish of chemotherapy-induced nausea would overcome me. After writing in my journal, it was time to turn off the lights and rest.

Chapter Eight
A side-bar on interdependence.

We've covered a lot of ground already. Some big ideas to get your head around. We've talked about this disease being in your body but nowhere else. We've talked about it not being able to touch your soul. We've talked about exercising some influence over its effect on your body with your mind. We've talked about relying on others to help with the stuff outside of your mind.

When we're in the best of situations, we often require the help of others. Certainly when we're in the thick of treatment and very vulnerable, it's reasonable to suggest that we might need more of that help. It might conjure the idea of "Dependence."

In western culture we place a great deal of emphasis upon the opposite of that idea: independence. We celebrate its importance in our culture. We honor it, we glorify it, we practically worship it. We celebrate the icons of that independence. We even have a national holiday recognizing its importance to our national psyche by recognizing the bold, important steps our founders took to establish independence from England. But it's really a myth.

Our celebrated independence is really not independence at all. Hold on to your hats, I'm not going communist or anything, just bear with me. It's really inter-dependence isn't it? Aren't we really celebrating our ability to handle most of our own stuff BUT with the help and cooperation of a great deal of people? Are we saying that we relied upon each other to stand on our own? Isn't that really life?

Now, right this moment, you may be relying - to a greater extent than you're used to - on the assistance of other people. But you're doing something for them too! Your allowing them to help you. You see, in order to feel good about ourselves, psychologists have shown that we must feel a connection to something outside of ourselves. We must feel a sense of belonging. It also helps us feel as though we are worthy of good things by doing good deeds. These feelings of belonging and worthiness are key components to our self-esteem. Additionally, helping others helps us feel good about our abilities. If we're good enough to take care of others' needs then we must be good enough at all of our other stuff to have enough talent left over to help out. This feeds our sense of self even more. By opening your life to others' help, you are providing these people with very important elements of their self-esteem. It's o.k. First of all, you'd do the same if the tables were turned and God knows, life throws enough at us, you'll probably get your chance. Second of all, if they thought about it, they'd be grateful to you for giving them a more personal source of this energy than simply writing a check to a local cause. Right now, you're not only a local cause yourself, but a deeply personal and highly connected one. Helping you is the best kind of help these people can give.

So, celebrate your interdependence. What's today's date? Write it on the line below.

_____

Today is Interdependence Day!

I declare a national holiday. We've got to work and we won't get any extra pay, but we'll observe the national holiday anyway!

Now, in the chapters to follow we're going to cover a lot of specific "hows" in the process of exerting influence over your body through your mind. There are a lot of exercises that you'll be doing. Some of the people around you might think you're on some kind of new age kick. Hell, who knows, you might be. I do know this, I'm convinced beyond convinced, I'm certain beyond certain, I know in my bones that these principals – along with the careful application of modern medical technology - saved my life while allowing me to maintain a great attitude throughout all of the pain and nausea and, yes, suffering.

I was willing to celebrate my interdependence out loud. I got a lot of funny looks. It's o.k. I was enjoying myself despite my misery and I didn't care what people thought. If you're happy, will you care what people think?

To help you get these ideas to sink in and also to help you in enlisting all those around you (your family, friends, miscellaneous visitors, caregivers, doctors, nurses, etc.) in your heroic struggle against negativity and to garner the strength and passion and enthusiasm of the universe in support of your healing, I've included the following page for you. Tear it out and hand it to your doctor. Photocopy it and post it on your door. Make a pile of them and give them to your visitors. Do whatever you have to do to make sure that everyone you know is on board with your new approach.

iCanSir!

Welcome to my living space.
It is a place where I've chosen to heal.

The good news is that no matter what happens to my body,
my soul will always be perfect!

I am committed to focusing on my desired outcome so that my mind will assist my body in receiving from the universe all that will help and block that which will not. I believe that this will be the key to my healing and that's exactly what I intend to do. I intend to heal. You can help!

You can help by:
> Keeping pity at bay and hope alive.
> Not discussing my diagnosis or asking about "chances" or the details of my treatment.
> Allowing me to discuss that which I want to discuss.
> Bringing positive energy into my living space.
> Reaching out to the great power, that great energy that exists within me and summoning that energy to assist in my healing.
> If you must do the opposite of these things, please help me by not doing them anywhere near me.

For instance:
1) For my doctors: I encourage a healthy professional dialogue and even debate among educated and trained peers regarding my diagnosis, treatment, even potential outcomes but I insist that to the extent these transactions radiate negative energy they take place far away from me and certainly are not to take place in my living space. You can help by conducting your professional skepticism out of my earshot. I have chosen you because I am confident in your professional abilities to garner the technical resources to help me heal. I have faith in you and ask you to have confidence in yourself. To help us foster this certainty as a team, Positivity, Confidence and Certainty will guide the tone of our transactions in my living space. I am grateful to you for considering this for me. Deeply grateful.

2) For my loved ones: I encourage you to research the disease that may have temporarily taken residence in my body. I understand that this may be a natural inclination. But since I am in the process of healing, I would like to minimize the very mention of it in my living space. You can help by choosing the words you use to express your opinions and thoughts regarding what I should do very carefully. Please, you can really help me this way. I am grateful to you for considering this for me. Deeply grateful.

Chapter Nine
What does nothing look like?

I promised that you'd learn tools. I promised I'd show you real actions that you can take to work constructively toward your healing. As you've no doubt surmised, the practice of meditation was an important part of my recovery and has been an important part of my life. The ability to separate the mind from the body and elevate our thinking to another plane, a higher level - if for even a moment - helps us capture important perspective. A key part of this process is the ability to get into alternative emotional, mental and physical states. This will make it possible to achieve higher levels of mindfulness. Higher mindfulness will help you find and liberate that true tiny voice inside. This voice will help you understand the universe and your place in it. I know that's a tall order but until you've meditated and experienced the information that you will be exposed to as a result of it, you really aren't in any position to argue with me.

So, higher mindfulness. How do we get there? Getting into a state of openness to inspiration does not require you to be an expert. Contrary to what you may think, it is not an experience reserved for gurus and swamis, or for that matter, rock stars or hippies. It's easier than you might think. In fact, anyone can do it. My kids can do it. I can do it. You can do it. If you doubt it, that's o.k. I will show you. For starters, know this, if you can breathe, you can meditate.

Try this for starters.

Read this through and then try it. Or better yet, tell a friend you've got to try something that might save and/or change your life and ask them to help you do this crazy thing. They'll help. If not, and you're in the hospital, ask someone there to help you. If that doesn't work out for you, visit my website, www.GeorgePKansas.com and order my guided imagery tape/cd. It's cheap and it works! If THAT doesn't work, try the short streaming version on the website for starters absolutely free!

First, get your body in a position in which you can be as aware as possible (i.e.: upright) AND as comfortable as possible. The idea is that you should be in a position where you're not likely to fall asleep BUT if you were to fall asleep you wouldn't have to do anything to hold yourself up. I don't want you falling asleep and falling off your bed. How would that look? I can hear it now. "Yeah I was trying this new relaxation and meditation technique, I fell asleep, fell off my bed and broke my nose!" That's not good for my business.

Seriously, you want to get your body in a comfortable position that you don't have to work too hard at staying in. I like to kneel on the bed or sit "Indian style" leaning slightly forward. When I kneel, the soft bed lets my knees sink in and I can keep my body upright which allows my breathing to flow nicely. You'll try many positions and find what's best for you. Remember, there is no <u>wrong</u> way.

O.K. Comfortable? Good.

Now, with your eyes open begin by drawing three breaths. They don't have to be particularly deep breaths. Just draw 3 regular breaths with just that on your mind. Just 3 breaths. In and out. In and out. In and out.

Nicely done. See, nice and easy.

Next try the same, but this time, make them real belly breaths. A truly deep belly breath is one in which you draw air so far down into the lobes of your lungs that your belly sticks out. If you can, draw these breaths through your nose. Belly breaths are more effective in bringing about the relaxation response if drawn that way. So if your nose isn't stuffy and you can do it, try drawing these next breaths in through your nose.

⨝ iCanSir!

Most people think that a deep breath is most effectively evidenced by one's shoulders rising. Although shoulders rising might be an outcome of a deep breath, it probably isn't. A true deep breath is evidenced by the displacement of your internal organs by your lungs filling with air and the diaphragm being drawn down into your lower body cavity, thus your belly sticks out. Some people call this belly breathing. Now you know why.

So, take three more deep belly breaths, this time watching your belly to make sure you're doing it right. Try keeping a hand on your belly so you know how doing it right feels. Breathe in through your nose. Let the air draw way down deep. Notice how your hand on your belly moves outward. Hold it for a second, and then let it out real slowly through your mouth. As you exhale through your mouth, try pursing your lips a bit as you might imagine a flutist would hold his/her lips over the mouthpiece of a flute. In through your nose real deep, out through your pursed lips. Notice how your hand moves inward as you release your breath from deep within you. Try this 3 times.

Niiiiiiice.

Now close your eyes and do it three more times. See why I told you it would be helpful to have someone read this to you!

One... Two... Three... Nice.

What crossed your mind just now? Nothing? A thousand things? Crazy things? Did you "see" a bunch of things that you have to do? A bunch of bills to pay? Your messy house? Your sister or brother you haven't spoken to in too long? Did you see other loved ones? Your doctors and nurses perhaps?

Jot those things now just to get them off your mind. Once they're written, you don't have to worry about them. You may come back to them later if you want. Get them out now so you can try to think of nothing in the next exercise.

_____

_____

_____

_____

_____

Next, draw ten belly breaths with your eyes closed. This time, try to picture what nothing looks like on the inside of your eyelids. If it helps, try to imagine a movie screen at the front of your mind. I know it sounds funny to suggest trying to imagine nothing by imagining a movie screen, which is decidedly not "nothing". That's why I said, "IF it helps". Ideally, just try to imagine the empty, vacuous nothing. Perhaps what outer space might look like. It might be void of all color, it might be all colors blending together. It might be black, it might be white. It might be dark, it might be bright. (Sorry about that Dr. Seuss moment there.) Nothing is probably a bit different for everyone. If you're using the movie screen idea, with your eyes closed, try to imagine what nothing would look like projected onto that screen. Once you get that non-image down, simply get rid of the movie screen.

Once you're capable of imagining what projecting nothing onto nothing doesn't look like, you'll have figured out how to imagine what nothing might look like. That sentence was designed to make your face crinkle and hopefully, after that, smile.

O.K. now it's time to draw those ten breaths with eyes closed imagining your non-image of nothing.

One – breathe a nice deep breath in through your nose, hold it for just a moment, then exhale through your pursed lips, nice and slowly. Niiiiiice.

Two – In with a nice deep, deep breath through your nose. Hold that for one second and then exhale nice and slowly through your gently pursed lips.

Three – Inhale and feel the nice, calming air fill your lungs with rejuvenating energy. Hold that wonderful energy in for just a moment. Now exhale nice and slowly and allow your body to release tension, negativity and stress.

Four – In nice and slowly. Hold it for a moment. Out nice and slowly.

Very good. You're doing great.

Five – In…Hold…Out…

Don't look now but you're meditating. You're doing wonderfully.

Six – In nice and easy. Hold that for a second. Out nice and easy.

Seven – In through your nose. You can feel the positive energy coming in and circulating throughout your body and consciousness. Hold that positive energy in there for a second. And out through your lips, nice and easy.

Niiiiice.

Eight – In. You're feeling the wonderful healing energy of the universe flow naturally into your body, bringing nourishing air and powerful ideas with it. Hold that wonderful healing power within you to give it time to transfer to your cells. And exhale the old air, the information you no longer need, the negative. Release it to the universe to transform for you.

You're doing wonderfully.

Nine – In. You feel the healing energy enter your body as it begins its magic transformation. Your cells are changing and improving and healing as you breathe. You hold it for a moment to allow your cells to nourish themselves. And you exhale the stuff you no longer need. The old ideas, the old way of thinking, the old you.

Beautiful.

And Ten – Nice slow deep breath in as you breathe in gratitude and healing and strength. You hold that wonderful healing energy in for a moment as your cells transfer what they need. And exhale ever so slowly and gently through pursed lips as your body releases forgiveness and stress and pain and negativity for the universe to transform on your behalf.

Niiiiiiice.

You're doing it. You're meditating. Your mind is creating gentle but powerful transformational messages and images that will enable your mind and body to work together toward your healing. Your mind is sending powerful signals to your cells to cooperate with the new images and transformation that you're asking for.

Your cells don't know the difference between what your conscious body "sees" and "knows" and what your mind "sees" and asks for. So, with your mind, through meditation, you ask for and create the images that you want your cells to adhere to. Health, Wealth, Peace, Prosperity, Healing, Energy, Gratitude, Forgiveness, Success, Balance, Love. It's all there.

Would you like to take it a bit farther? Let's take it a few steps farther, shall we? This time I'll take you down a path that worked wonders for me. At a time when I was told I had no bone marrow left and that until my body saw fit to replace it (or I borrowed it from someone else – ouch) I would have to rely on transfusions of blood to keep me alive, these images allowed me to begin the process of replacing my bone marrow. Eventually, I required no further transfusions and no surgery. In just five months, I was on my way to having replaced my bone marrow to the point where I no longer required treatment or medication of any kind.

Continue to draw the deep breaths but now we're going to focus less on the breathing and a bit more on something else. I want to ask you to imagine the location of the source of the cancer in your body. Where do you imagine it to be? Two things might help but are not necessary. One is to know a little about your disease. Two is to know a little about the biology of your recovery. It might help if I give you an example:

I was diagnosed with Leukemic Reticular Endotheliosis. The nickname for this disease is Hairy Cell Leukemia because the lymphatic cells that have gone hay-wire - the issue that characterizes this disease - look like tiny black fuzzy tennis balls under a microscope. I knew from my research that my problem was being caused by these crazy white blood cells taking over and preventing my healthy blood production. The little terrorist buggers were occupying the parts of my body that are used to produce my blood. I had learned that this is done mainly in one's pelvis, spine and hands (not the long bones as I had once learned).

So, I imagined the deep recesses inside the bones of my pelvis. I imagined tiny narrow conference rooms with very low ceilings. I imagined these characters sort of hiding out in there, well-armed and shabbily dressed. I imagined them somewhat well-organized but not terribly mindful or motivated. I imagined two stem cells (the good guys). The only chance my body had to make my own, healthy blood.

My last hope. I imagined them hiding out in the duct work waiting for their chance to exact their revenge, capture the hairy cells and begin to make my blood again.

All the while breathing deep, deep breaths, I imagined my stem cells having conferences.[17] I called them my healthy cell conferences. I called these conferences to order often during my month long stay in the hospital. I am convinced that these very vivid visualizations empowered my body to make the necessary changes in body chemistry and create the appropriate biotic environment to manifest this visualization in reality. Yes, of course the chemotherapy and medicine made it possible too. But I say to you with equal certainty that the fact that I saw very clearly what I needed my body to do, played a key role in manifesting that reality in my life.

Let's take it even one step further. You can do what I did next. Still breathing deep, deep breaths. Nice and easy. In and out. In through my nose, holding it for a second and then out through gently pursed lips. I imagined that deep within the recesses of my body, I maintained what I called my Situation Room. Yes, just like the one in the White House!

In my SitRoom I held conferences with my Joint Chiefs of Staff. These were all of the healthy cells, stem cells etc., that I could muster from the far regions of my inner space. I would also call secret meetings in the late-night hours. To these meetings I would invite "ninja cells" and "cleaner cells". These cells were secretly charged with stealthily hunting down my leukemic cells, destroying them, packaging them discreetly and disposing of them without a trace. These were my special forces.

I know that it's a bit dark and ironic that a peace loving, tree hugging, meditator like me would yield such violent metaphors for healing.

---

[17] At this point, I imagined just two cells conferencing together. I was in such bad shape, I imagined only two little guys left. Gods among microbes!

Hey, remember I said sometimes healing gets ugly? This was one of those times. Sometimes the images are peaceful. Sometimes they're downright nasty!

They were microscopic mercenaries sent to do my "wet works". There was a catch, however (and this is where the irony is evened out a bit). Immediately prior to "liquidating" these undesirables, the mercenaries were sworn to deliver a final, two-part message to these troublemakers. Immediately prior to termination, the mercenary cells were to say to their intended victims, "Thank you, you're forgiven."

As if to say, we appreciate what you've taught us, we grant you absolution for the harm you've done, but you're no longer needed or welcome here." Ahhhh, emotional congruence. Kharma. There is balance in the universe.

Now, while breathing peacefully and enjoying the peace and calm that comes from the deep, satisfying belly breathing, try that imagery. See what crosses your mind. Take notes. If you come up with imagery that works better for you, jot it here. Also, please let me know what you come up with. Others may benefit from it. You can email me at gpk@georgepkansas.com (please put "meditations" in the subject line).

_____

_____

_____

_____

_____

_____

It may take some time to get the hang of this. Be patient with the process and be patient with yourself. If at first, all you can do is sit still for a minute, well then that's a minute longer than you meditated yesterday isn't it? Whether your meditating on forgiveness or wellness or peace or absolution or fitness or weight loss or weight gain or red blood cell production, you've got to stick with it and accept the tiny little triumphs. Each moment you invest reaching for a higher mindfulness is a moment that you glimpse into eternity. Given the road we're traveling together right now, I can't think of a better investment. NOT because you're preparing for that "eternity" thing any more than I am right now. But because we ALL need the energy that encompasses eternity in our corner. Right here and right now!

Keep in mind, this is something we could all do more of. It's something that I hope you'll continue to do for years to come. Years from now, if you're paying attention, you'll continue reaping the rewards. Hopefully, you'll do less and less stuff that you'll feel guilty about, but still the meditating is going to be good for you. Hey, the Catholic Church has been advocating confession for absolution for centuries. Although I don't believe a priest is more qualified than I am to dole out "holy" dispensation, I think the Catholics were at least onto something useful here.[18] The idea of regularly getting "it" off your chest is right on the money.

Here is another little side note that relates to my personal beliefs. You don't have to believe this way for all of this stuff to work. It's just my point of view. I respect that you may differ. In fact, I embrace those differences even when it may be inconvenient for me. I urge you to try to do the same. While I respect people's faith, I get frustrated when leaders take advantage of their institutional power and pervert that faith at the expense of the believers. Personally, I feel that your soul and my soul are as much a part of God as any living

---

[18] I should probably mention here that I am what I've heard described as a 'recovering' Catholic. I was raised attending Catholic church and have since found my own path for spiritual development, nourishment, etc. I don't espouse any path. I believe that is for everyone to decide on their own.

organism. As such, I believe that we can all, with practice, communicate just fine with "him/her" without the intermediary of a priest or other officiant who claims to be more in tune with God than you or I. I feel pretty confident in our ability to tune in on our own. I'll concede that we don't all do it often enough, but I believe we have the ability.

Additionally, I resent the implication of some religious leaders that I should have to subjugate myself to another human being for the privilege of a direct line to God. I think that line is right there within us at any given moment. As I said, however, the basic idea of appealing to the higher power for aid in the forgiveness of others and the self-forgiveness of our own transgressions is a sound one. If it leads us to a higher level of spiritual mindfulness and compassion and peace, then I'm all for self-reflection and forgiveness.

I wrestled with the question of whether to include this insight into my own beliefs out of concern that it might cloud your view of the beneficial information the book has to offer. Ultimately, I decided to give you more credit than that. I'm choosing to believe that if you're reading this, you've opened your mind to new ideas and that you respect the possibility that there may be other plausible interpretations of God that can coexist along with your personal beliefs without infringing upon your ability to believe what you believe. Just as I acknowledge that your interpretation is just as right as mine as long as neither of us hurts one another or infringes on the other's right to believe what we believe. Fair enough? Onward!

The point is that making an ongoing effort to renew your spiritual account by honestly accepting responsibility, learning your lessons and then releasing the mistakes, makes a lot of sense. It's good for your soul, and it's good for your body too!

I've said before that the cancer is me. The cells that are problematic are my cells. If I harbor deep feelings of guilt and negative energy, those cells will be poisoned, and something will go wrong. If I make amends for those things, learn from them and take steps to assure that those harmful things never happen again, then I may forgive myself and move on in higher mindfulness. If I forgive myself, my cells – by extension – are forgiven as well. I can also go directly to those cells and forgive them outright.

There are two essential sets of metaphors that can be employed here. Those two sets of metaphors are 1) death and hatred and anger and war on the one hand and 2) life and love and forgiveness and peace on the other. Between the two, the first one is the most common cited in the cancer experience as I've seen it and how it had always been presented to me prior to my experience. Think about it. "I'm gonna fight this one to the death!", "I'm not giving up until I beat this thing!", "I'm going to poison my cancer and kill it before it kills me!". Do these sound familiar?

As I was thinking about healing, my treatment, chemo, recovery, etc., I was thinking, "If this cancer is me, do I really want to heal myself by hating me?" It didn't make sense to me. In fact, when put in those terms, given my new insight, it sounded like that would indeed make matters worse! It sounded as though if I thought about hatred, anger and judgment, since hatred, anger and judgment are what made me sick, then those thoughts would just trap me in "sick".

I decided to change the traditional approach from one of anger and violence toward my cancer to one of love and   forgiveness.   I'm certain it made all the difference. I know it sounds a little crazy to tell someone to "love" their cancer. And I guess it is a little crazy, isn't it? I'm really not asking you to love your cancer though. I'm asking you to love yourself enough to not hate your cancer. There's a difference. It may be a subtle one.   Subtle differences, I think you'll agree, sometimes can make all the difference!

To describe my condition and my plan to people, rather than using expressions including words like "kill", "destroy" and "battle", I said things like "I forgive my cancer.   I'm grateful to my cancer for

94

teaching me what it was meant to teach me. Its work is through and it's free to go now." I would meditate to my cancer cells "You may die now. I no longer need you. I will not mourn you as I heal myself. Healthy cells of mine die everyday and I do not mourn their passing. They die as a natural part of my body's renewal and so shall you. Upon your death, I shall be renewed as I always am. Thank you. You're forgiven." That was one of my favorites.

Write a good one for your cells now. Write one – or at least the rough draft of one – that you think might tap into some of that forgiveness and gratitude for you.

_____

_____

_____

Of course, you're more than welcome to use mine!

You'll notice throughout this book that I often went back and forth between the different metaphors. Violence in one reference and peace in another. The reality is that they both can work. I've said it many times that life is full of paradox. They coexist. The duality of life is strange. The bottom line is that they are both effective at different times and sometimes they're effective at the same time. Just like in life!

These affirmations were remarkably effective in constantly buoying my emotions while the chemotherapy continued to work toward reducing my cancer counts in my body. Together, my mind and modern medicine eliminated my cancer and I remained happy and positive and certain all the while! As sick as I got, as painful as it was, as many times as I just would have rather not gone through it, the whole experience was a joyful one. One of a great many lessons that shall shape my life. Hopefully, for years and years to come.

Chapter Ten
What does life mean to you?

If you desire - truly desire – to make a quantum improvement in your condition – if you want to live, truly live - then you'll be willing to risk some new behaviors to accomplish it.

> "If you're not actively involved in getting what you want,
> you don't really want it."
>
> Peter McWilliams

Life.

What does that mean to you?[19]   Jot some thoughts now on what exactly Life looks, tastes, smells, sounds and feels like.

_____

_____

_____

_____

_____

_____

At this moment in time during my personal struggle, I had written in my journal what this meant to me. Again, my journal entries appear in this font.

_____

[19] This is not exactly the same question as "what is the meaning of life?" is it? I guess maybe it is. Did you know you had the answer all along?

Winning the fight. Thriving throughout the battle. Feeling whatever pain may be necessary but not allowing the pain to distract me from the joy, peace and balance that love and real life can bring.

For the duration of this book, I'll be referring to all that this means to you metaphorically as "survival". The essence of this reference is really creating an emotional and psychological environment in which you actually enjoy the process of, well, fighting for your life!

I decided when I was in the hospital that – live or die – my stay in the hospital was going to mean something. I was going to have an impact. Even if it was as simple as giving helpful feedback to the many doctors, nurses, interns and medical students who would poke and prod at me during my stay. I also decided that I would approach my illness as I had always approached my wellness. That life was simply too uncertain all the time to let an opportunity to learn, grow, teach, and enjoy myself slip away.

Now, I didn't know how nauseous I was going to get. I didn't know how tired I would get. I didn't know how much hair I'd lose. I didn't know how much weight I would lose or gain or how much pain I'd be in. Had I known ahead of time, it may have been harder to make such a commitment to enjoy myself. I'm certain that I still would have made it though. I guess I just believe in the immortal words of Abraham Lincoln that echo in my mind:

> People are about as happy or as miserable
> as they make up their minds to be.

I've always decided to be happy. At least to always find the lesson or the positive in every experience. I've never regretted it. It helped me survive. My advice to you is to do the same. There is NO downside.

iCanSir!

The commitment I'd like you to make before going much further - without getting too crazy – is to believe that…

<u>you can experience psychological adversity,</u>
<u>physical and emotional pain and injury,</u>
<u>and still - without kidding yourself - be mindful of spiritual</u>
<u>joy.</u>

Experiencing pain and being mindful of joy at the same time! My hope is that this idea will be something you come to believe in so strongly that you'll apply the principals set forth in this book to many of the other important areas of your life for years to come. I've seen lots and lots of people do it and believe me, it is so very worth the investment of time, money and pain!

I learned a lot more about this when I began running marathons after my recovery. Although going through chemo was far worse than running a marathon, I did learn a thing or two about enduring pain. Chemo didn't hurt my knees. Running does!

You'll see as we work through this together. My sister Elaine advised me with characteristic wisdom to read Jumper Cables for the Marathon Runner's Soul - my first book. I followed the program I had laid out in that book. I followed it to the letter. What's funny, odd, unusual about that is that I followed the guidance of a book I had written for marathon runners. The wisdom I had borrowed from business and shared with athletes and the wisdom I had borrowed from athletes to share with business turned out to be uncannily accurate for the healing survivor!

It blew me away that the lessons I had laid out for runners training for a marathon applied to my situation in the hospital. For this reason, with only minor modifications, these pages follow the same general path as the corresponding section in the marathon book. I explain that because I don't want you to get upset with me if you ever happen to read the marathon book and think "well gee he just cut and pasted the meat of the book". Well I didn't. I've reviewed every word and rewritten those sections with specific parts to apply exactly to those areas where battling for your life and working toward healing diverges from preparing for a marathon. As I say, it's almost scary how infrequently that happens. But it does happen, and when it does, I've addressed it with the powerful stuff I came up with while battling my own battle.

When it doesn't, it's not because I was lazy, it's because the message from the original text fit so perfectly that it was counterproductive to change it. My objective is to share my message to help you deal with whatever it is you're dealing with. My purpose is to actively do my part in changing the vocabulary of survivorship. I've carefully chosen every piece of this book to further that mission.

I'm going to shift your perspective a little bit. I'm going to get you to look not at the evidence that proves you'll be miserable or you're going to die (one could do this all day but it won't aid in your survival), but rather at the evidence that proves you can survive and maybe even enjoy the ride!

In fact, many people would just as soon convince you why you can't do it. That's what the world is often best at. It's the way they were conditioned. They just never made the conscious adult choice to change their perspective. What will help you survive, however, is your attitude. What will help you beat the disease will be your willingness to accept that success is a reality and there exists every reason to support this conclusion. In short, what will heal you (among other things) and do it with a smile on your face and in your heart is certainty in yourself!

"The greatest pleasure in life is doing
what people say you cannot do."

Walter Bagehot

Working as a Results Coach (results oriented life-coach), I have known the great pleasure and honor to witness many of my clients attain personal successes which clearly support this conclusion. Here are some of the clues which I've observed. I encourage you to ponder your own successes as you work through this book, as your healing progresses and as you witness your own victories (however tiny they may appear to be). As you prepare for this peaceful battle, know this:

1) You're capable of anything. You've probably heard this before. I've read it a thousand times in Napoleon Hill's writing: "What the human mind can conceive, it can believe. What it can believe, it can achieve!" This, of course, includes your healing.

2) If you are reading this right now, you are a survivor of incredible spirit and determination. There is an ancient oriental saying that the journey of a thousand miles begins with just one step. You've demonstrated that you can take that first step by either purchasing this book or seeing your doctor or undertaking a regimen of healing of some sort. You've demonstrated that you can follow through. Now it's time to take it to the next level.

3) You are not the first person ever to be diagnosed with a life-threatening illness. You may be the first to have survived the particular illness with which you're dealing. Many others may have laid a clear path for you. There are thousands and thousands of stories of people who have beaten cancer of all sorts and other diseases of all sorts. If they can do it, so can you. If others haven't done it, it doesn't mean that you can't be the first. You can. Thousands of people before you have fought this fight and won. Thousands of those people have reported actually enjoying the process. Although it may be hard to believe, some of them have

even done it with greater obstacles to healing than your own. They have done so under worse conditions, harder times, with less resources. There is no reason whatsoever that you could give to justify not trying it, which would be more credible than any reason that justified their having done it.

4) In the final analysis, we all will die. None of us knows what, when or how our end will come. You and you alone, will ultimately bear the power, the responsibility and opportunity to respond to each and every moment anew, as though each moment was dropped into your life fresh, with no judgment, no predetermined path, no outcome carved in stone. While very little of what happens TO us is under our control, very much of what happens WITHIN us is. So very much of our lives is, in fact, subject to the influence of our own mind!

You have chosen a path toward this healing that may include health care practitioners, complementary therapies, etc. You must KNOW that you and your team CAN heal you. While working through this book, you'll KNOW that you're also mindful of joy and gratitude and peace the entire time.

No matter what happens to my body,
my soul will always be perfect.
No Matter What!

A quick note on your path to healing (medications, treatment, diet, etc.) In my research I've uncovered hundreds if not thousands of resources and thousands of ideas for approaching a particular disease and healing. I know that for every patient and survivor, there is a different philosophy that governs their healing. For this reason I don't advocate any one particular approach, philosophy, pharmaceutical, or diet for you. I am certain that no matter what approach you take to your healing, this program will complement it. I can't imagine a situation in which having a positive, peaceful, confident, joyful, gracious and grateful attitude wouldn't help. Can you? Honestly?

As far as doctors and hospitals and medications and nutrition, I'm leaving that for you to decide – as an individual, as a patient, as a survivor. As I made the assumption earlier that you'd like to enjoy most of this process, I'll further assume that you are doing the homework you need to do in order to identify a treatment and recovery protocol that is appropriate for you in addition to the techniques in this book.

If you don't have a plan, talk with your caregivers. Seek out support. If you absolutely don't know where to start, please visit my website – www.georgepkansas.com - click on "Health Resources" and that may help you get started. The information is out there. In most cases, you're not going to be reinventing the wheel here. In some cases, you may be treading in uncharted waters. It's o.k. You'll be a pioneer. What you learn will help you and many others.

The balance of this book is set up to support you in your healing for three weeks (21 days) for starters. It's been said many times that the human neural nets are so succinctly wired, it takes as long as 21 days to break an old habit and restart a new one. This book is designed to help you replace unhealthy ideas that are probably unsupportive of your healing and replace them with proven, positive, healthy ideas that most certainly will support your efforts toward healing.

Since this book in its many incarnations started out as a sports training book for marathon runners, and since that book served me so very well as the foundation for my thinking during my recovery (and again and again as a marathon training book) much of the workbook portion will use sports references, quotes, stories, etc. to support the information and exercises you'll be presented with.

I wasn't much of an athlete really when I read and used this information. I was hospitalized and could barely walk up a flight of stairs. That condition did not stop me from benefiting greatly from the wisdom in the sports quotes and stories I read. You don't have to be an athlete for this information to touch you. I knew it when I wrote it for the runners but became certain of it when I used it myself. Runner or not, athlete or not, you'll benefit from it too!

"You have to expect things of yourself
before you can do them."

Michael Jordan

Now you've got a plan. You've outlined with your caregivers a detailed plan to approach your illness with confidence and begin the healing process. Decide to have faith in that process. I know it's scary but if you don't decide to have faith in it, it's going to be that much harder. The folks who crafted it know what they're doing, right? You chose them and this plan for a reason. So, you have good reason to believe it will work. You're plan is - or will be - consistent with the plans that have allowed thousands of people before you to heal and get better and move on to do the great things they're meant to!

As you implement this healing plan, you will experience many things. You may, as I did, become sicker at first. You may, as I did, experience all manner of discomfort: pain, nausea, dizziness, hair loss, vomiting, diarrhea, mouth sores, muscle aches, blurry vision, you name it. Your plan will have you suffering, to be sure.

That suffering – coupled with this book - will separate you from the folks who strive for wellness and remain miserable the entire time. That suffering will be your rite of passage. The book is your road map. There will be times when you'll catch yourself laughing while in absolute agony. You'll recall a funnier time of your life exactly when you need to and instantly, your demeanor will shift. You may continue to be in discomfort but you'll do so with a strangely confident and oddly joyful way about you.   It may confuse you, perhaps, but you'll be grateful for it.

As each day passes, as each discomfort is experienced, as each of these pages is turned, you will be closer to your dream.

Remember our mantra, "No Matter What!"   We're starting with the next 21 days for now. You must get through the next 21 days enjoying the path along the way. 21 days of joy, beauty, inspiration, pleasure! Of course, overlaying this is the same 21 days of possible pain and sickness. In order to accomplish the task of being mindful of joy and gratitude during this experience, you simply must experiences these days in a state that   averages   the mindfulness of those ideas that bring you these feelings.   You may not be mindful of these feelings the entire time, but if you are awake 12 hours of the day and 31 out of 60 minutes of every hour is invested in mindfulness of these positive emotions, then when averaged out, you've been mostly positive. You've maintained an 'average constant mindfulness' of those ideas that bring you positive emotions. Simple – perhaps. Easy? That may, of course, be another story. But hey, as I'm fond of saying, "If it was easy, everybody'd do it!" With this book, you'll be ready!

To use a sports analogy, in order to be able to say that you enjoyed the experience, you must maintain an average mental "pace" of joy. Just as if your goal was to break a certain time in a race, you would have to maintain a "pace" of "X" in order to break that time. The question, therefore, isn't "Can you run a mile in X minutes and Y seconds?" Of course you can. The question isn't "Can you do this for every mile or every minute of every day?" You don't have to. Just as you'd need only to average X minutes and Y seconds per mile for your goal, you need only average a mindfulness of joy for each of the next 21 days.

You can do this. I know because I've seen it done! I know because I did it! I know because I do it everyday. If I can do it, you can do it!

How? This you accomplish through your conditioning.

"My grandmother started walking five miles a day when she
was sixty. She's ninety-five now,
and we don't know where the hell she is."

Ellen DeGeneres

Follow your program. No excuses, only reasons. It's your life. No one is going to read this book and do the exercises for you. Even if you have someone reading this book to you, you're still going to have to be the one to do the thinking. Embrace it. Each time you do, you bring yourself closer to your dream. If you don't do something – a step you already decided was necessary – at least be honest and recognize that you didn't do it because at that moment you either wanted to do what you did instead, more than what your plan said to do or (and you only get to use this very sparingly) you simply couldn't do it because you were unconscious. Why you do this, only you will be able to tell yourself.

At risk of sounding like a broken record, I want to restate that this stuff is important no matter what your situation is. None of us knows how much of our life we have left. We can almost universally agree, however, that regardless of HOW MUCH life we have, we all want to be sure we maximize HOW we live that life. Correct? You've heard the expression, "It's not how many days in your life that's important, it's how much life in your days!"

This program will help you put life in your days. No matter what! Following your program won't be a problem for you. To insure this, however, you must make two lists.

The first of the two is a list of at least five <u>negative</u> consequences of your failing to follow your program. Five painful things which you will experience if you don't meditate on a given day or if you fail to follow through with your program in some way. I mean, this is 21 days for crying out loud. I know you may be in rough shape right now, but hey even in the shape you're in you can give this a try for 21 days. Heck, you can stand on your head that long! Although I don't advise it in your condition!

Seriously, I know you may be feeling pretty horrible right now. I remember, <u>very</u> vividly, my days in the hospital. Especially those first days. If you're conscious, and even remotely able to, I'm encouraging you to please employ this program daily. You'll get the most out of it that way!

So, back to the list of potential consequences of not following the program. This was my list while in bed in the Bone Marrow Transplant Unit:

Death

Disability

$$$ Trouble

Dependence

Physical Limits

What's your "If I don't do it" list look like?

1) _____

2) _____

3) _____

4) _____

5) _____

The second list of the two, is a list of at least five <u>positive</u> consequences of your following your program, sticking with it and enhancing your mindfulness of enjoying the process of life. This list will serve as a constant reminder of just what you're fighting for!

This was my list:

Life

Strength

Ability

Joy

Wealth

What's your "When I'm doing it" list look like?

1) _____

2) _____

3) _____

4) _____

5) _____

If you can get to one, or have a friend get to one for you, do this on a computer because 5 copies of these lists must be distributed in five different places: 1) On your bathroom mirror. 2) On your desk. 3) On your car dash board. 4) On your refrigerator and 5) On your night stand. Now, when I was at this point, I was in the hospital with no real hope of getting out anytime in the next month or so. So I just wrote it on the workbook and looked at it a lot! You certainly can do that too. If you are out and about, though, take advantage of the different settings in which you can reinforce your reprogramming efforts. Remember, those neuro-nets are pretty hardwired. This means you've got a lot of reprogramming to do. The more opportunities you create to chip away at those old neuro-nets, the better you will get at maintaining your mindfulness of joy, gratitude and grace.

> "The past is history, the future is a mystery,
> and this moment is a gift."
>
> Deepak Chopra

It's not called the 'present' by mistake!

Another important step in the process is to evaluate regularly. Measure your progress. In order to gauge your small successes along the way, you must measure your progress. Inside this workbook you'll find occasional progress sheets for you to use to tally your daily improvements. Additionally, every other page in the workbook is a journal page. Jot whatever thoughts come to mind. <u>What</u> you write doesn't really matter nearly as much as <u>that</u> you write some thought, some impression, some feeling each day. Keep in mind that everyone will have their own measurements and standards to strive for. For me, during my stay, we were constantly monitoring several things which told us a lot about my condition: my hemoglobin count, my hematacrit count, my platelet count, my white blood cell count and my temperature. These measurements were what told me how I was responding to treatment. For this reason, we kept track of everything relating to these factors. Seemingly constantly! At all hours of the day and night, these factors were gauged and recorded.

You'll measure a number of factors of your own for your journal, as you'll see. You'll keep track of how you felt during your day. How you're feeling (physically and emotionally) on that day generally. How your eating has gone that day. How your breathing felt. Also, should you ever – upon your surviving this challenge – forget what has happened to you and how committed to this process you are at this moment, this information will be very handy in getting you to knuckle down and do what needs doing to heal yourself! Lest you should ever forget!

Remember, what's worth living is worth recording. This way you'll be able to look back and evaluate what you did and how it helped or what you might change to improve your approach. Regularly, you'll measure your factors. For now, jot a list of what might be your factors? What might you measure so you'll know how your body is responding to your efforts to heal? If you don't know, you need to ask more questions!

_____

_____

_____

_____

_____

_____

Why keep track of this information if you're not going to be open to adjusting your tactics, right? By keeping track and being mindful of this type of information, you'll be able to make necessary adjustments in your approach. Be it a simple visualization or a dramatic change in your program, you'll now have the information at your fingertips to make these important decisions.

Listen to your body. The millions and billions of cells in your body have the collective inherent wisdom to tell you what you need to adjust. For instance you may feel fatigued from pushing yourself to stay up to date on returning correspondence. This fatigue may begin to have an effect on your hemoglobin levels. This may tell you to

109

adjust your activities to accommodate more rest, for instance, or increase meditation, or reading or social support. Listen, your body will talk! Listen, then, record. Pay attention to what those images look like and record that as best you can. Be attentive to how those adjustments make you feel and make notes of those feelings.

Learn as you go. As each day's events and experiences accumulate and each bit of data is collected, you'll be gaining valuable insight into your condition. The more you listen to your body, the more information you have and absorb, the more you prepare for your dream. Remember when I asked you to write what "Life " meant to you? That's your ideal. That's what you're shooting for. Your body and mind work in concert. You cannot optimize one without utilizing the other!

> "Once you are physically capable of winning a gold medal,
> the rest is 90 percent mental."
>
> Patti Johnson

Throughout this program, you'll be asked to do some thinking. To maximize the benefit which you derive from centuries of thinking before you, you'll be asked to integrate some new ideas. You'll be challenged to really push the limits of your comfort zone (if you haven't already). Taking care of your mind may be something which you've overlooked in the past. O.K., perhaps not overlooked but I'll bet certainly under-thought.

You may have less experience in conditioning your mind than you have in conditioning your body. You may have overcome other challenges without concentrating on conditioning your mind. You're shooting for a quantum accomplishment this time. This challenge, let's face it, is unique.

This workbook will help you recruit your own mind to help in your conditioning process. Your health challenge is not just a physical challenge. You probably know this from your experience. As you train your mind, your body will be assisted and strengthened too. If you haven't enjoyed this phenomenon in your experience, for now, accept that this is so and wait for the evidence.

Your mental conditioning at this point is at least as important as - if not more important than - your medical regimen (meds, radiation, chemo, diet, etc.).

No Matter What!

Quantum improvements (big improvements) – over time – in mind, body & spirit, are the big payoff. You've identified exactly what those benefits are. You already remember why you want this. Quantum improvements require you to be willing to push your comfort level way out. Remember…

When you can't, you must.
When you must, you can.

You'll have to try some simple but very effective (and proven) strategies. This rest of this book will help you to…

Keep a journal
Try new mental games to improve your meditations
Remember your compass (<u>why</u> you're fighting the fight)
Stay tuned in, connected & supported
Stay psyched
No Matter What!

In short you're going to train your mind as well as your body. You're going to do something you may not be used to doing. You're going to learn to become more mindful. You'll be more mindful of the condition of your body. You'll be more mindful of your emotional

iCanSir!

states. You'll be more mindful of the effect your attitude has on your performance, your health, your overall sense of balance.

iCanSir!

Chapter Eleven
How to use the rest of this book.

The idea behind this is simple. Your mind – like your body – needs to be trained for maximum performance too. The good news is that this is possible. A hundred years ago, we knew very little about what we could do to train our minds. Now we know dramatically more about it.

Each page of this book will correlate with a day along the path. Each page is broken down as such:

1)   The day. Day 1, Day 2 and so on. We'll start with the first 21 days. It takes 21 days to start a habit so we're shooting first to change the way you think and create positive habits. After that, you can get more pages at my website, www.georgepkansas.com. If you can't afford to buy them, send me an email and we'll get them to you anyway. I want you to have this information more than I want your money.

2)   The quote of the day. These will generally be hinting at the strategy for the day and usually be either witty or inspirational or both. I hope you like them because we dug up thousands of them and I'm please to have assembled such a collection. The really crazy thing about these quotes is that somehow, as if by magic, the quote of the day always just seems to be the perfect quote for whatever you happen to be thinking about that day. As I've mentioned, when I was in the hospital, I used my first book, *Jumper Cables for the Marathon Runner's Soul* ® as my guide. It always struck me how uncanny it was that I had assembled these quotes years before and each one was exactly what I needed to read on the day I read it while dealing with my Leukemia. For this reason, I have changed very few of the quotes from the original collection.

3) No Matter What…! Just reiterating the mantra for this challenge! Remember the rest of this mantra…"No matter what happens to my body, my soul will always be perfect!"

4)   Daily Strategy.   The text on each page will give you your "homework" for the given day. You may occasionally see me refer to you as an athlete. It's not by mistake. In some instances, what you're going through makes you - well – an athlete! Why not recognize that?

In some cases, the stuff I'll have you do might be a reach. On other days it might be a piece of cake. For a runner we'd want to have a daily objective that was doable and measurable. In your case it may be that. But it might also be something less immediately measurable. The idea, though, is to raise your mindfulness. In your situation, that may be more important in the short term than a specifically measurable thing to do. On a given day, your task might be simply to meditate for twenty minutes.   Specifically measurable and doable, right? It might be, however, something a bit less measurable or even a bit less doable, like simply increasing your mindfulness of a particular idea, like the fact that your message, your gift, your special energy is important and worthy and noble. The specific measurable part of that might simply be to draft an affirmation and repeat it ten times throughout the day. The cool part of this is that as you revisit this down the road, these tiny accomplishments will serve as important inspiration for reaching for a higher ground!

The process that you are about to embark on and move through will utilize what we've learned about training our minds over the past 80 years or so. The most profound and effective method of training our minds is a simple and obvious but very neglected process. It's been called associative and behavioral conditioning.   It's been called programming and self-hypnosis. It's even been called brainwashing. All it really is is talking to yourself in such a way and with enough consistency to form positive thinking habits. That's it in a nutshell. Positive thinking habits.

ℛ iCanSir!

Throughout the work pages – or later on in the supplemental exercises - you'll see that I refer to certain "Modalities". Don't get thrown off by this if you've never used this lingo before. A modality is really just a fancy way of referring to one of your amazing senses. Traditionally we think of them as Touch, Taste, Smell, Hearing and Sight. Some people are mindful of a famous "sixth sense". This sense is sometimes credited for influencing others' behavior. I happen to believe in the sixth sense because I know my daughter uses hers on me all of the time!

There are really three modalities that I'll mostly use throughout this book to help you strengthen your mind/body partnership for the challenge you're now faced with. The one you'll probably come to rely on most often is Visual or sight. When I mention the Visual as the day's target modality, I'll be trying to get you to "see" something. It may be as simple as noticing what the weather is like or what people are doing, etc. It may be more complicated in that I'll ask you to "see" yourself doing something during your recovery or treatment. This visualization skill is critical and you'll develop that skill as you work through these daily exercises!

Another modality we'll use is the Kinesthetic modality. This is your sense of touch, balance and movement. Your sensitivity to the condition and needs of your body is one of the most important senses you can fine tune. This skill will be sharpened throughout these exercises too. It will serve you well not only during your treatment but throughout every area of your life, as well.

The last modality we'll really get into in this book is the Auditory modality. This, of course, is your sense of hearing. Sound can play a major part in keeping you inspired to move ahead during your "training". If you're not sure of this, turn on the soundtrack to the movies, Chariots of Fire, or Rocky, or any other music that has a rousing crescendo to it and observe if you don't get excited and inspired to do something.

As you become more aware of these modalities, you'll get better at using them to your advantage. There may be times when you say to your self, "he's got to be kidding me". When those times come, just do it anyway and don't give me any grief about it. Trust me. This works. Remember, I've seen it work! I wouldn't suggest you try if I didn't know it worked. Remember, it won't do you any harm and it can ONLY help! I'll discuss ideas such as developing visual strategies or using auditory stimulation or appreciating your kinesthetic sense. Together, you and I will train your senses in each of these areas by conditioning each of them repeatedly, over time.

6) Finally, I'll finish each day by inserting my personal notes from my experience in the hospital or immediately after. As I mentioned, this may help you appreciate that you are not really alone in this. Right this instant, there are lots and lots of minds thinking thoughts very similar to yours. Tune into them and you may feel a little bit less alone, a little bit stronger, a little bit more hopeful!

My grandmothers used to talk to themselves.
I think they were experts at psychological conditioning!

When you start to see the habits forming, you'll start to see your performance changing too. What will start out as small improvements will serve as tiny reinforcements. Small physical signs that your "new" mind (really new "mindfulness") is working. Your friends, family and caregivers should start to notice too!

You may notice that a handful of these strategies are repeated as you work through these 21 days and onto the pages which follow as you download them from the website[20]. These are the most effective strategies. They'll be the most helpful to you in accomplishing your goals.

---

[20] Do I really need to say it again? O.K., O.K., www.georgepkansas.com .

Often readers and folks who have attended my seminars have reported that as they begin seeing these changes they also become more "mindful" of positive changes in other areas of their lives too. These strategies have helped thousands of people to improve their physical performance just like you. Athletes such as Andre Agassi and Michael Jordan. Performers such as Tina Turner and Christopher Reeve. Many people I have worked with have had results similar to those of these "stars" using these same principals with my guidance. Clients ranging from amateur golfers to professional fighters, marathon runners and professional football players! And don't forget my most direct testimonial, my own personal experience!

These people have all employed these strategies to improve the quality of their thinking in order to manifest positive changes in their lives. Why? Because it works. It works because it depends on nothing else but the most mysterious, powerful and reliable system in the world. Your own mind! Good luck. I'm cheering for you!

> "My mother taught me very early to believe I could achieve any accomplishment I wanted to.
> The first was to walk without braces."
>
> Wilma Rudolph

Wilma Rudolph was the first woman to win Three Olympic Gold Medals in none other than Track and Field. She overcame obstacles. Sexism, racism, Polio, poverty. Wilma's example needn't only be appreciated by women or people of color. Male or female, we've all – at one point or another – felt the sting of adversity. Make a list of some of the "obstacles" that you've overcome in your life. It should make you proud to remind yourself that you, too, have made more of yourself than your circumstances may have indicated at any one time. Take a moment to feel that pride. What are you thinking?

This was my list: Skiing, College, Law School, Politics (34th District), Divorce, Custody (10 yrs), now Cancer

What adversities have you overcome before this?

_____

_____

_____

"Follow your instincts.
That's where true wisdom manifests itself."
Oprah Winfrey

At the end of the book, you'll find Appendix A. Appendix A will help you do and redo those wonderful lists you've dabbled in. You'll even do a bit more of them as you go through the first 21 days. I can't say enough about these lists. They are what has kept me focused on my dream, day in and day out, for over 20 years. I have not given up because at the very moment when I could have feared my death the most, I was calm and collected and as focused as ever on what was most important to me. Beyond that, the deep sense of peace and empowerment that I felt in that moment when I realized that my life carried very little regret, was priceless. I attribute that sense of peace to the clarity that these lists have given me over the years. Do the exercises, you'll be so very glad you did.

You're about to embark on the first 21 days of a new life of empowerment, clarity, certainty and confidence. After that, you'll read about how my life shaped up after my cancer experience began and some of what I've been up to since. Beyond that? Who knows? I hope you'll keep in touch.

iCanSir!

Day 1

"I wake! I'm grateful for this glorious day!"

George P. Kansas

**No matter what happens to my body,
my soul will always be perfect!
No Matter What!**

Earl Nightingale said "Success is the progressive realization of a worthy ideal." Whether you define success as a total remission or a better understanding of your health, your success will be judged by no one but yourself. You will judge your success upon how you travel along the path. When you train your mind as well as your body, when you improve as a patient, as a caregiver or as a survivor, when you grow as a person, you succeed! As you progressively realize this valuable experience (one step, one page, one victory at a time – literally!), you experience success!

Each day you'll keep careful track of your performance states. This will be crucial to training your sub-conscious mind to regulate your "mental pace" at one of positive mindfulness of joy, beauty and gratitude. Over time, this WILL happen. Each day, you'll record your mental states on the appropriate day's page. You'll be asked to record your thoughts, feelings, etc. about how you feel on a particular day. That's for your eyes only. You may appreciate being able to come back to that information another day. This will sharpen your mindfulness skills.

Let today's be to just complete the day's exercises and start your journal entries!

iCanSir!

These are notes from my hospital stay:

****

PIC line today? Start Chemo?[21]

****

Start with writing how you define success?

Success =

_____

_____

_____

_____

_____

_____

---

[21] Remember, these are my notes that correspond to these days in my journal as I worked through the same exercises you will. This "pic" line (Percutaneous Intravenous Catheter) was a medical appliance that consists of a long tube inserted at my elbow and worked up through my blood vessels into my aorta just atop my heart. This allowed my chemotherapeutic agents to drip directly into my heart and therefore disperse faster throughout my body without the risk of "burning" the particular spot on my arm or specific blood vessel where the chemo agent might ordinarily be injected. Ingenious. Gross, but ingenious! The spot where it was inserted in my arm can still be seen. It's a scar I look at often. It reminds me of what I've overcome. There's a positive in everything. Even something as simple as a scar the size of the head of a pin.

Keep in mind that today, you may have a slightly different idea of success than you may have had three months ago. And even what you may have three months from now. That's just because you didn't read this book six months ago! Don't worry. It's o.k. to be saying to yourself "Hell, today, success means keeping my eyes open for another hour. Hell, today success is making it to tomorrow." That's o.k. If you had read this book six months ago, you'd have included that in your definition anyhow. Your perspective would have been better aligned to begin with. It's not your fault. Maybe I hadn't finished the book back then.

My personal notes (remember, these will always appear in this text style):

****

Notes from Robert's (dear old friend from modeling days) visit with Anthony (dear friend from law school).

Robert's quote in response to my passing gas (sorry, yes, even cancer patients fart!)

"quando u kooloo sauna, ah persona si sente buona!"
"When the ass sings, the person is feeling good!"

Anthony's prayer.

"Father we know your hand is in it.

℞ iCanSir!

Help GPK so that he may share his blessings with many people!"

My meditation to my hairy cells.
I thank you for what you've taught me, are teaching me or what this experience will teach me. I forgive you for damaging my body, for what you did to my bone marrow, blood & spleen.

Success: Waking up, staying up, breathing, exercising, loving the kids, loving family, working, making some dough.

Fight first doubts – medical residents using language like "well probably" "usually" blah, blah, blah when referring to the appropriateness of the chemotherapeutic agent being used in me.

Lesson: When you have a credible positive and a credible negative...go with the positive everytime!!!

****

What credible, positive information do you have about your condition?

_____

_____

_____

What things are you grateful for today?

_____

_____

iCanSir!

How is today a glorious day?

How are you going to measure your progress? White blood cell count? Red blood cell count? Markers? Talk with your caregivers about what will serve as reasonable indicators of your improvement.

Of equal importance are some of the non-"measurable" indicators of your improvement. Energy, lack of pain, attitude, skin tone, etc. Ask your caregivers to tell you if these are likely to show change as you improve. Do they have scales against which to measure these "un-measurables"? Learn a little about those. Become an expert at observing!

ℝiCanSir!

Journal Entries

_____

_____

_____

_____

_____

_____

_____

_____

_____

_____

_____

_____

_____

_____

_____

_____

_____

_____

_____

_____

_____

_____

_____

_____

_____

Day 2

"I can do it. I'm sure I can.
I can. I Can. I CAN!"
Anyone who ever did anything worthwhile!

No Matter What!

You must be absolutely sure of yourself. You must realize and accept that all of these strategies that you are employing were employed in some measure by those who've faced these challenges before you. When you need it most, you will have that confidence! For now, trust the universe to provide the resources you'll need to accomplish this important mission!

Remind yourself of the reasons you want to renew yourself. Remind yourself of why your health is important to you. Remind yourself of the reasons being well means anything to you at all. Remind yourself of the benefits you will experience by staying mindful of the fact that No matter what happens to your body, your soul will always be perfect! No Matter What!

****

My first day of chemotherapy.[22]

****

---

[22] I swear I wrote this book two years before I even knew I had cancer. The quotes were tiny little, perfectly timed gifts from the universe. I mean, I was starting chemo today. Look at that freaking quote! "I can do it!" I am certain that my mind planned for that day nearly two years before when I started the marathon book. Tell me there's not at least some kind of sense to the idea that all time exists at any moment.

It's just crazy to me that 2 years or so before I needed it, I wrote this reassurance to myself in the hospital. "I can do it!" It's something we should be telling ourselves far more often. We should be saying to people everywhere, even when we "know" it can't be done. Mathematically, the bumble-bee can't fly. It's body is too heavy and it's wings are too small. Fortunately, the bumble-bee isn't a mathematician. The bumblebee doesn't "know" it can't fly. It just flies! How much of what we don't do is prevented because we "know" it's impossible? What if we "knew" it was possible? What if we didn't think so much about what we "know"?

How do I feel today?

_____

_____

_____

_____

What does that look like?

_____

_____

_____

_____

Take a look at some of my journal entries from this day.

****

I felt a bit dashed by something the resident said yesterday and it's still sticking with me. He used words "probably", "usually", "pretty sure", and "not a classic case". The more I think about it, the more it pisses me off. Tomorrow, I will read him the riot act. I mean, if we're "not certain" of my diagnosis, then what the hell am I pumping this poison into me for? As far as I'm concerned, my head doctor knows what I have and he's treating me for it. If he says I've got X, then dammit, I've got X. I'm taking this Cladribine to treat Hairy Cell Leukemia, not because the labels go well with my eyes! And I'll have none of this "usually" nonsense. Cladribine cures the thing. Period! Jeeez.

I woke up today. I feel strong. It's a great day to get up and take advantage of the opportunities the world has to offer.

I am grateful. I forgive my cells & myself. I am strong. I am healthy. I let the unhealthy cells die without mourning them and my body is renewed.

Flesh/Blood – I will talk with the resident about confidence.

Beginning of a funny speech. Stage is dark, the voice comes on over P.A. "Patient presents with complaints of shortness of breath, chest pains, associated with large muscle exertion, normal activity symptom free, however blood test reveal pancytopenia. Bone marrow biopsy resulted in dry tap. Tissue sent to Cytology/pathology for screening. Diagnosis: Hairy cell leukemia. (I don't recall what was supposed to be funny about this.)

I feel fine. (suuuuuure you do!)

****

iCanSir!

Journal Entries

Day 3

**"A nail is driven out by another nail.
Habit is overcome by habit."**

Desiderius Erasmus

No Matter What!

If you're used to doing something a certain way, and the old method has become habit for you (you've done it the same way over and over again) then you're probably getting the same results that you're used to getting. The key to obtaining quantum change is to try different strategies. Different strategies often yield different results. When you come across a strategy that yields better results than the ones you've been getting, stick with it for a while. If it becomes a habit that serves you, go with it. As it serves you less, try another strategy. Maybe even try another strategy after a while anyway. Just to stay sharp and expand your comfort zone. Keeping track of your health factors (vital signs, blood values, etc.) and states may seem foreign to you now. As your mind becomes more comfortable with being aware ("mindful") of your mind's and your body's "pace", it will begin to regulate your body's actions to bring them into congruence with your goal. Your body will "learn" how to heal in order to manifest your dream of health and vigor! Pretty cool, eh?

****

Stay positive. Force yourself to meditate.   √

****

"Rrrrrrrrrepitition is the mother of education." Said Dr. Sanford Van der Hyde (my 9th grade German teacher).

♀iCanSir!

In order to train your mind, you must inundate it with new ideas over and over again. Just like you learned vocabulary in high school, you must teach your mind a new language. The language of your dreams.

Take 10 sticky notes. On each, write "No Matter What!" in the center of the note. Underneath that, write a big juicy "YES!" on them.

Stick them everywhere!

These were some of my journal entries.

****

Stay certain!!! Certainty beats a full house and a Royal Flush.

Scrambled with the help of Jill Hughes (a hospital volunteer), found radio just in time to hear Jeff and Brian on Roundtable. Yesterday I did an interview on WGY in front of two med students. John and Chris who were here to practice their physical exams. Alex before him. Monday I had two physicals too. Jyoti was in charge of those two. Well done. Tarik and Samir.

It's all good. Rock2Rebuild Tsunami Relief Concert tomorrow!

Good name for a program..."Cure yourself silly"

****

iCanSir!

Journal Entries

Day 4

"Concentration is the ability to think about absolutely nothing when it is absolutely necessary."

Ray Knight

No Matter What!

You know, sometimes in all the excitement of our day to day "getting it done", we get distracted from some of the really important stuff. We get caught up. We keep putting off and putting off those tasks that seem "unnecessary". In fact, some of those things are unimportant, unnecessary. Some of them, however, - sometimes the ones we put off the longest – are very beneficial to us. Did you ever put something off and then finally do it, only to say to yourself "gee, had I done that originally, I would have saved myself a lot of aggravation"?

Take some time – maybe a half hour or an hour – and invest some time for yourself. Just yourself. Schedule this "appointment" for yourself right now. Take that half hour or hour and just be. Put some music on and meditate on your life, the people you love, the things you've done that you're really grateful for. Maybe do this in the bathtub with the lights down and some candles burning. Give yourself permission to just relax.

How do I feel today?

_____

_____

_____

℞iCanSir!

****

Meditate to music.   done

total relaxation is difficult but possible. 90 degree supination helps. (sic) Music helps but not critical.

Breathing is key!!!

****

Peace is a choice. Today – in every deliberation - choose peace. Remember the story of Chicken Little She ran around the barn yard screaming "the sky is falling, the sky is falling." Guess what? The sky isn't falling! If a Chicken Little comes along, simply say to yourself, "I'm not buyin' today! NEXT!" and choose peace.

Aaaaaaaaaaaaaaaahhhhh!

****

Journal entries: I've awoken. Today's going to be a great day!

Kevin (my old friend, former law professor and divorce lawyer): "So...will the hair on your balls fall out?" on speakerphone, just as a nurse was walking into my room! I thought I was going to pee I laughed so hard.

Stephen B. (dearest friend from law school)- "GPK, don't worry, if you need a bone marrow transplant,...my wife will be on the first plane to Albany."

My niece has pledged $50 of her money to Rock2Rebild to support Tsunami relief! Some of the best news all day!

9:30 PM. Rock2Rebuild * is well underway. My cell phone rings.
GPK: "Hello"
Brian Kaplan (BK): "Hey George,?"
GPK: "Hey Brian"
BK: "Hey, I've got a few thousand people here who want to say hello!"
GPK: "Hey Albany, how's everybody doing?"
BK: "One, Two, Three..."
Crowd: "Get well soon, George!" roar!
BK: "O.K. hold on." Then Brian put the phone down and played "Hopeful"[23]

Many good feelings of accomplishment. (I cried myself tears of joy until I fell asleep this night!)

****

Surely there are some things that you can look back on with great pride of accomplishment. Even the tiniest little victory, today, can be reflected upon as heroic. Think of a couple of those things now.

_____

_____

Good way to end the day today…

_____

[23] One of my favorite songs. Available on Decaffeinated at www.yodelingloonrecords.com

iCanSir!

Journal Entries

_____
_____
_____
_____
_____
_____
_____
_____
_____
_____
_____
_____
_____
_____
_____
_____
_____
_____
_____
_____
_____
_____
_____
_____

Day 5

"Today I'll allow myself to simply become."

George P. Kansas

No Matter What!

I hope you can imagine the peace I felt as I wept those tears of pride while falling asleep that February night. While the fruit of our collective labor of love touched the lives of thousands of people, I slept having had a glimpse of what my legacy might look like.

It doesn't have to be big to be a great legacy though. Have you ever heard that expression "you may not be someone special to the entire world but to someone special you are the entire world"? It goes something like that anyway. The point is that you have to know that you don't have to have done anything that has made what you consider to be a global impact in order to feel good about leaving a legacy. The legacy you leave often will be unknown to you anyway. For many of us, much of that legacy will blossom long after we're gone. The ideas we leave behind take shape through the efforts of other people. The impact of those ideas shapes the future. That's what a legacy is.

Because it happens in the future, we can't force it in the now. Like much of our successes, we must simply allow it to happen. I'm not advocating sitting back and just letting the world pass you by. I'm advocating the pursuit of your dreams and letting your dreams meet you half way. Besides, right now, things are a little different. A little. Because you may be in a situation where being "out there" hustling toward your dreams isn't an option for you everyday due to your health, I'm going to have you concentrate first on getting your "house in order". First we're going to work on knowing what those dreams are in the first place. I like to say that we're humans becoming not just human beings. We become a little bit more each day. We're not handed a road map or design specifications for our life when we graduate from kindergarten. The path we take must be discovered as we go. We need to learn to allow that process to be and at the same time enjoy the paradox that it is also true that in order to manifest our truest intentions we must take those affirmative actions that we're inspired to take.

****

Busy day, visits, law stuff, meditate

Actual: Chilled but good walks outside and with kids

****

What would you dare to do if you knew you would not, could not fail? Invest one minute to write non-stop to answer this question…

_____

_____

_____

What would you dare to do if you knew you would not, could not fail BUT you knew with 100% certainty that exactly 3 years from today you'd be struck by a bus and killed?
Invest one minute to write non-stop to answer this question…

_____

_____

_____

♀ iCanSir!

What if you sat on the edge of your bed one day, today, and were certain that your time would come to an end any day? What would you look back on the past 90 days and wish you had done?
Invest one minute to write non-stop to answer this question...

_____

_____

_____

Tough love question for the day...Why haven't you done these things already?

Seriously, think about the real reasons these "Edge of the Bed" items remain undone... Invest a minute or two to articulate those reasons.

_____

_____

_____

Are any of them any good? Good enough to let even another day go by without doing something, ANYTHING, toward accomplishing them?

How many of these Edge of the Bed ideas involve either saying something to or doing something with another person?

If experience with my audiences is any guide I'd bet my shirt that your Edge of the Bed list contains at least one item that involves either saying something to or doing something with another person or other people. Perhaps it just showed you that you'd like to take more time for yourself.

� iCanSir!

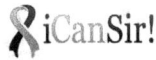

Regardless of what it exposed for you, this list - this digging and sweeping - uncovers and illustrates things that, in the recesses of your mind, are very important to you. My advice is to really look at those reasons why you may not have done these super-important things yet. Acknowledge that your life just got in the way and commit to yourself that these things are now just too important for you to let go even one more day.

Imagine all of the emotional energy that will be freed up as a result of doing these things. Imagine how much higher the other items on your list can now go, now that you've got the really important stuff under control.

This can be a profoundly emotionally freeing experience. Don't let the sun go down on the day today without taking some serious action to make these things happen.

****

Again, I awake. Today is a good day! To heal, to grow, to connect, to love. Today is not just a good day. Today is a glorious day!!!

I talked with "Fred" (one of the patient service guys) today about the music business. According to Fred the keys are 1) Desire, 2) Work, 3) Networking, 4) Appeal to market. This kid is smart!

I am the luckiest man in the world. I think I know what Kirk Douglas meant when he said "My stroke of luck"[24] I just feel lucky, fortunate, grateful, grateful, grateful.

---

[24] You've GOT to read this book! www.georgepkansas.com/readinglist

Just came back from a walk. I headed to the "M" entrance which is the beautiful crescent entrance. Ran into Steve M. from high school. He works part time at the airport handling luggage. Great bennies. I asked if he thought there'd be work for an able bodied cancer survivor? He said to call him. I will. [25]

Came upstairs!!! 4 flights. I kind of bound up the last one. A bit winded and dizzy but felt great. Dr. P saw me in the hallway. She could tell I was smiling behind my mask. She said "you are the healthiest person in this hospital!!!"

****

Like Nike says, "Just Do It". They say it because it sells sneakers. It has in fact sold more sneakers than any other single slogan. It does more than that, though. For millions of people – from athletes to zipper salesmen - It works! It inspires people. It transforms millions of people from mere <u>consumers</u> into <u>evangelists</u>. Nike devotees proclaim Nike's benefits to anyone who'll listen. They visit Nike Towns across the globe just to tune into the Nike energy. We can take a page from the Nike book and use it in the training of our minds.

By telling ourselves, "Just Do It!" we can jumpstart our psyches. By using "Just Do It!" as a self starter we can trigger ourselves to take action where we might not ordinarily do so. By taking that first step, we set in motion the parts of our bodies and minds which create momentum. Just Do It! Turn this page and keep reading and writing your journal entries.

---

[25] As it turned out, later that year, when I was well enough to work again, I did call Stephen. I ended up working for the airline for a full year. In addition to getting in great shape from carefully loading your luggage into the bellies of planes ;-) I enjoyed many free trips both with my kids and on my own.

iCanSir!

The first step, the second step, the third step. Before you know it, you've forgotten what was holding you back. You've begun the process of forming a new habit!

How about those measurable indicators? How are they doing?

Indicator: _____   Indicator: _____

Status:_____   Status:_____

Notes:

_____

_____

_____

These measurable indicators are important but they are not everything. Remember, the path and the goal are only parts of the bigger picture. How we respond to the things that happen along the path toward our goal is something else. Probably, in the long run, those responses are even more important. So, if your body is responding positively, great. If it's not happening as fast as you'd prefer, that's o.k. Focus your mind on what is improving. What about those intangible, non-measurable aspects of this experience? How are you holding up emotionally? Spiritually?

Meditate. Find what there is to be grateful for right now. In this very moment.

_____

_____

_____

ℛ iCanSir!

Journal Entries

_____
_____
_____
_____
_____
_____
_____
_____
_____
_____
_____
_____
_____
_____
_____
_____
_____
_____
_____
_____
_____
_____
_____

Day 6

"Achievers are those people who get done, all of those things they don't have time to do!"

GPK

No Matter What!

You may think of a thousand other things that you need to accomplish today. If you're having trouble "squeezing in" your time to meditate, think of this…

Imagine how it will feel when you hear the words "you're in remission". Imagine what it will be like to wake up in the morning and not dread a chemo treatment, transfusion or injection of some sort. These are the types of sensations that people who are "well" don't have to even give a second thought. We are the lucky few, however. These thoughts, therefore, must cross our mind. Having to think about this stuff, however, makes us stronger. When we can force ourselves to go there in our minds, we confront a strange demon. One that not only reinforces our will to live and live well, but also helps us muster the energy to wrestle this disease to wellness.

Take the time to imagine what those sensations will be like. Ask yourself, "How will it feel in my gut to be in remission?" "What will those words sound like?" "What will a deep breath feel like then?"

Feel that now. Hear those words now. Breathe that breath now.

Meditate. Just don't have the time? Make it. Remember, no excuses, just reasons. Schedule it! Do it and then write the journal entries!

Either you're part of the solution or part of the problem. Today, be part of the solution. You pride yourself each day in being a problem solver. It's what makes you good at what you do. How often do you give yourself credit for that, though? Today, be mindful of the good things you've done for people. Make a list if you have to. Not just stuff that you've been paid to do, but stuff that you did which was "above and beyond the call of duty." Stuff you didn't "have" to do, but did anyway because it was the right thing to do. Go ahead. Write five things down that you did that fit that description.

_____

_____

_____

At the end of the day, be the one who was part of the solution more often than not. It strengthens the character and the mind. As your mind and body strengthen together, your mind/body partnership becomes stronger.

****

Just some thoughts today. Give blood. Donate. Volunteer. Open mic. Rock2Rebuild. These are things I've done during my life to help others. That energy is coming around and saving me now!

One of the nurses, Tony, scared the s*#t out of me last night. It was hysterically funny. I was having a dream that I was taking a shower with Christy Brinkley. It wasn't particularly erotic but it was the first time in several weeks I even had the energy to think about a girl, a naked girl! I was sleeping and dreaming and Tony came in to wake me for my meds changes. He was whispering my name over and over and my ears could hear him but my mind wasn't registering it. Until he touched my arm to wake me. I must have jumped a foot off the bed.

I explained the dream and we both laughed so freaking hard I was crying.

****

It turned out to be a running gag for us during the rest of my stay. He would buzz me on the intercom from the nurses' station and say "George, this is Christy, can I get anything for you? Some soda, some candy, a hand-job?"

Pretty freakin' funny at the time. Remember, it's cancer. It's not pretty, but it can be pretty funny.

****

A little metallic taste in my mouth today. This morning. Weird.

Tired today. Visitors. Wow I'm lucky. Tired today. Sleeping all day pretty much when not visiting.
Headache now for third or second day.
Nauseous today for really 1st significant time. Temp. gradually climbing up a degree at a time. Now 100 or so. Admin. Prophylactic broad-spectrum antibiotics "just in case".

Very tired.

****

iCanSir!

Journal Entries

Day 7

"It feels good to have so much to lose."
Gwyneth Paltrow's character 'Rosie' in <u>Shallow Hal</u>

No Matter What!

If your entire life went smoothly all of the time, how would you really know when things were going great? If you look around to see how much you've got to lose, you'll no doubt count your blessings. Be grateful in this very moment to have known such abundance. In case you're wondering if you fit this description, trust me, if you're reading this book, you've known abundance. Right now, no matter how bad you may think you have it, someone, somewhere, has it worse. I KNOW that this is a hard thing to grab onto sometimes, especially now. I know it because I was there, right where you are.

When you're depleted, when you feel you really have it bad you'll need something to jump-start you. Please don't feel inferior for feeling it. Everyone does at some point in their lives, a given year, a day. Music is one of the most powerful means of locating this jump-start for many people. Your auditory faculty (your hearing) has been proven to be one of the most sensitive senses relative to its impressionability. For our purposes, this means that you have the ability to associate sounds powerfully and with relative ease. We'll put this to work for us. If you've ever dated and had "a song", you know what I mean.

What songs do you know that have the ability to stoke you up the moment you begin to hear them on the radio? Today, think of a play list. A list of songs that have been, or that you think would be, inspirational to you. Write some of those titles here. We'll come back to this.

---

iCanSir!

For now, just imagine your own private concert comprised of your dream list of artists, performing your dream list of tunes specifically for the sole purpose of pumping you up. If you can, compile – or ask someone to compile – the actual songs on a disc or tape for you.

****

Night of nausea but Phenergan (sp?) helped & slept like a rock. Woke up, sat up, feel grateful. Perfect timing for today's message. It could <u>always</u>, <u>always</u> be worse! Today's a great day to get better!!!

****

The night before I made this entry was the first night that the nausea really hit me. I mean I was buckled over in agony. Lying in bed doubled over and grasping my gut with both hands. I remember looking at the clock and it being around midnight and I couldn't fall back asleep for the life of me.

I was amazed at how uncomfortable I was. Suddenly I truly understood what I believed to be a fraction of what my mom may have felt when she was dealing with her chemotherapy. I remember that the nurses came in an encouraged me to allow them to administer an anti-nausea medicine. "It'll help you sleep" they insisted. I refused. Why? I have no idea. Well, that's not entirely true. You see, I'm very sensitive to any type of analgesic or anti-inflammatory medication. Even the smallest dosage of allergy medicine makes me loopy for hours. I really don't like that feeling.

Eventually, half in and out of sleep, it was too much. I was groaning in agony and suddenly an idea hit me. I started laughing with the affect of a complete lunatic. I said to myself (I can't recall if I said it out loud) "find the good in this Mr. Motivator!" (Remember from Chapter Four?)

The next time the nurses checked in on me I succumbed. I gave in and allowed them to give me their remedy for the nausea. In retrospect, I must admit, that being a hero was ridiculous. The Phenergan helped so well. I ended up sleeping like a rock. I think the reasoning that eventually got to me went something like this: In order to heal, you need strength. In order to be strong you need rest. You can't rest if you can't sleep. You can't sleep if you're nauseous. So, fight the nausea, take the remedy, sleep, get strong, heal thyself! Sounded good to me.

I guess the point of this is "hey, don't be all macho, if you can't sleep, try whatever the experts tell you it will take to get you your rest!"

iCanSir!

Journal Entries

_____

_____

_____

_____

_____

_____

_____

_____

_____

_____

_____

_____

_____

_____

_____

_____

_____

_____

_____

_____

_____

_____

Day 8

**"It's a requirement. And it may sound easy,
but nothing will be harder. It will test your head…and
your mind…and your brain…too!"**
Jack Black's character 'Dewey' in School of Rock

No Matter What!

I know that nothing about a marathon <u>sounds</u> easy. Doesn't look easy. Doesn't feel easy. I feel <u>un</u>easy just thinking about it! You may share these uneasy feelings. Whether you've run a race or not, the thought of it may cause you some stress. The same is probably true of whatever course of treatment that might lie before you right now. Chemotherapy, radiation, transplant, processing, complementary therapies, etc.

I know that when I was told I had to undergo 7 days of 24 hour/day intravenous infusion, I really didn't know what to expect. Hair loss, nausea, dizziness, fevers, sores, wounds, bleeding, diarrhea, you name it. The only thing I knew was that I was in for an endurance challenge. For lack of a better word, a marathon.

When my sister Elaine suggested to me that I read my own book to help me through my personal marathon, at first I just thought she was kidding. "Well, you wrote the book!" she told me. "No, seriously, you wrote the book. Literally!" she insisted. I got it! I asked the kids to bring me my working copy of the book so I could start "using" it.

The good news was that I knew it worked for runners. I figured it had to work for me. All of the principles are the same for an aspiring survivor as they are for an aspiring marathoner. The stakes are a lot higher, but the principles, I was convinced, are the same. I knew that the energy which was creating my dis-ease would now be called upon to inspire me for healing when the time came.

ℛ iCanSir!

This entire book is about preparing your mind. Your body – through the training you do to accompany this book – will prepare itself. It won't happen in a vacuum, however. The two are intertwined. Inextricably.

As you meditate, exercise and heal and as your body gets used to getting itself healthy, your mind will be paying attention. It will be taking notes on your capabilities, what jump-starts you, and what pushes you over the top. So, as you challenge your body, you'll be challenging your mind too. Pay attention to the observations you make. Take notes. Write them onto these pages.

What were you mindful of during your day?

****

In a word, exhaustion! I think of something Rick told me yesterday. I think he called them "The Four Covenants" 1) Be impeccable with your word. 2) Don't take anything personally. 3) don't assume Anything. 4) Always do your best.

My best right now is inside me. I visualize the speeches I'll make in the future.

Tired, tired, nauseous, nauseous.

****

It's funny that what you need, comes to you when you need it. The idea that my best was still inside me was somehow reassuring. It helped me not feel guilty about not working while lying in bed doubled over with nausea. It helped me realize that I was still capable of great things.

You may be frustrated that you're in this condition. It's normal. It's a part of the process. Your experience, however, can only transform your self image if you allow it. You need to feel competent and relatively in control in order to feel good about yourself. Everyone does. It's easy to feel out of control when you rely on so many other people for everything in your life including your life!

Try to shift your definition of what "being in control" means to you. I know it may be new to you. Try thinking of being in control not as manipulating the actions and events around you but more as manifesting your personal states in a way consistent with the inner picture of that which you desire. Try thinking less about what you want to "make happen" and more about how you feel and what you think about.

As you gain an aptitude for what we in the "inspiration/coaching business" call "managing your states" you'll come to appreciate that this is really the best way to manipulate those actions and events around you. By starting on the inside (which is all we really can change) we begin to exert influence over the environment around us. It just takes time and practice.

ℛiCanSir!

Journal Entries

_____

_____

_____

_____

_____

_____

_____

_____

_____

_____

_____

_____

_____

_____

_____

_____

_____

_____

_____

_____

_____

_____

Day 9

**"Make the most of yourself,
for that is all there is of you."**
Ralph Waldo Emerson

No Matter What!

What will be the measure of you?

When you are in remission and the struggle of your recovery becomes a bit less intense, however many days from now, how will your legacy be improved? Changed? Will what you stand for have changed at all? You may not be thinking about this experience as representing anything historic or significant or spiritual. If that's the case, that's O.K. No one said this HAS to be a spiritual experience.

In this world, however, the measure of us – like it or not – is reflected in our influence. Like it or not, we set an example, we make history, we create significance. Even if this influence barely extends beyond ourselves. Like the ripples in a pond, our influence – no matter how tiny we may personally perceive it to be – goes on and on.

****

Tired, nauseous
I hope my stay here has influenced the doctors and staff here.
Sleepy – 2 days now without answering my phone or opening my eyes for that matter.
Up at night just long enough to watch West Wing.

****

iCanSir!

Think about what and who you influence in your life. Think about that while you go about your day today. Throughout the day, observe your influence as it unfolds in front of you. What did you do? What did you say? How did you do and say it? What did that feel like?

Influence is a lot less about "pushing" an event than it is about inspiring the forces that manifest an intention. Often we imagine influence as making something happen or getting something done. We see it that way because the outcome is what we see with our eyes. The "real" results. Often, however, we exert our influence over things by merely thinking about them. Without being able to "see" changes, we still are able to bring about a change. Have you ever felt the need to speak with someone and a few hours later you turn a corner and run into them? Have you been asked by a friend to pray for them or someone they care about? Ever said, "I'll keep my fingers crossed for you?"

The point is that you've tried to exert your influence over something without actually doing anything other than think. You may not have been aware of it, but you've practiced the art of manifestation before! Exerting influence is about manifesting or making real an idea that we have a vision of. We have a picture in our mind, we want to make it real, we try to manifest it by exerting our influence over those things, people, events that need to occur in order to bring about the outcome we desire. That's what I mean by influence.

When you settle in at the end of your day, what observations can you make about events during your day? What role could your intentions have played in the events of the day? Write your reflections on today's Journal Page.

Go to it!

iCanSir!

Journal Entries

_____
_____
_____
_____
_____
_____
_____
_____
_____
_____
_____
_____
_____
_____
_____
_____
_____
_____
_____
_____
_____
_____
_____
_____
_____

Day 10

"They are able because they think they are able."

Virgil

No Matter What!

You may be just getting used to the idea that "thinking" you can do this, will actually make a difference. It may be your first conscious attempt at controlling the influence your mind can have on your physical performance. I say "conscious" attempt because I know you've done it before, you just may not have been paying attention. Have you ever talked to yourself - even for an instant - and said something like "you can do it" or "don't panic" or "just one more step and I'm at the top"? I thought so. It happens to all of us at one point or another. See, you're more experienced at this than you may have thought!

For some of my clients, this step – embracing the idea that thinking you can, makes it possible – has been the biggest step. If this is the case for you, it may help to look at it this way. What have you got to lose? If you're a skeptic, this is as good a time as any to deal with it.

What's the worst-case scenario? You try this whole mind-body thing for a few months. You undergo your treatment regimen in order to become well. In the meantime, you keep a journal about your "training". Also in the meanwhile, you read some entertaining quotes and maybe learn a thing or two about the psychology of performance.

Then, you either get well or you don't. That's true no matter what you do, isn't it? Whether or not you use this book and these principles. Worst case – your "performance" isn't any better than it might have been. You still have all of these personal reflections to look back on as you perhaps prepare for the next step in your battle or share your thoughts with other people in similar situations. Your worst-case scenario is that you've created valuable information. You've created a memoir of sorts that you can look back upon or use in upcoming chapters of your life. That's not a bad contribution to a legacy.

Now, I happen to believe this won't be the case. I <u>know</u> this stuff can't hurt and I'm 99.99% sure it will help.

The upside? We'll cover that tomorrow.

(Yes, yes, you can read ahead a little because I know you don't want to just ponder that stuff all night without a taste of the upside!)

This day during my experience was my mom's birthday.

****

Mom pledged to me 5 years ago on January 20 that she'd always keep an eye on us. I feel that she must be doing just that. I feel is an ethereal sensation to be sure but it's a feeling – a sense – nonetheless.

I spiked a fever last night, come to find out. I must have slept right through that temperature taking. I was pretty nauseous last night and the Phenergan rocked me pretty good. Today I woke up well though. Head was clear. Thought I'd go home but they need to see a few days of no fever. Get my blood back. It could be a few days more, as many as 10. It is what it is. No sense getting frustrated by it at this point.

And this is my favorite…

Been to hell, no reason to think the trip back would be just a walk on hot coals!

℞iCanSir!

****

Let me explain this a bit. First, in retrospect, you can probably appreciate the potential for frustration here. I've been in the hospital for two weeks at this point. I've been told I'd be in the hospital as little as three weeks or as long as six months. Every day, a different factor rears its head making the determination of when I'll go home impossible to predict. You can see that after a couple of weeks of that and being told 10 days more isn't that big a deal to me.

The hot coals remark is just my favorite. Ten years ago at a personal development seminar I walked across hot coals as a demonstration of my ability to control my mind/body state to avoid pain and damage to my body. It was an empowering experience I shall never forget and have used those tools every day of my life since then. I get a kick out of the fact that as I lie barely conscious, my sense of humor, hope and enthusiasm expresses itself with that golden nugget! Tomorrow there's another one.

🎗 iCanSir!

Journal Entries

_____
_____
_____
_____
_____
_____
_____
_____
_____
_____
_____
_____
_____
_____
_____
_____
_____
_____
_____
_____
_____
_____
_____
_____
_____
_____
_____

Day 11

"Keep away from people who try to belittle your ambitions. Small people always do that, but the really great make you feel that you, too, can become great."

Mark Twain

No Matter What!

O.K. The upside of all of this psychology stuff? The easiest way for me to demonstrate that this works is just to tell you a story. It's about an experience a client of mine had. She was preparing for the New York City Marathon and hired me to help her do this.

We concentrated most of our time for those several weeks on enhancing her mindfulness of gratitude. About 6 weeks before the event, she suffered an ankle injury and an old knee injury began to pester her again. She didn't think she'd finish the race this time around. She decided to lower her sights a bit and was determined to be satisfied - consider herself successful - if she were able to at least get to the "half marathon" point.

As she ran, she recalled the constant reinforcing we had done with gratitude. Everywhere she turned, with every step she took, she was reminded how good she had it. She carried with her the last page of her copy of the original Jumper Cables for the Marathon Runner's Soul ® book with her. Folded and carefully pinned to her singlet, it served as her reminder of all she had to be thankful for. Her mindfulness of gratitude propelled her to the finish!

Injured and in pain the entire race, her mindfulness of how relatively alive she was got her through! She called me from the finish line. In tears. She cried tears of joy, pride and gratitude that New York November afternoon! She sounded as though she had just been awarded the Nobel Prize! She was elated and joyful and there was a lightness in her voice that I just can't do justice to on these pages.

Her <u>running</u> didn't prepare her for that. Her <u>thinking</u> did!

Yours will too!

****

The mind creates a picture – the body makes it reality.

My Hairy Cells are now dead. They're forgiven and I'm grateful for what they've taught me. Now my mind sees healthy stem cells making healthy marrow, making healthy red and white blood cells. I see me healthy. My body will take it from here.

I visualized two stem cells meeting in my pelvis and heard the conversation they may have had. Divvying up the labor and being so cheerful in their work.

Thoughts. Although I may look like I wallow in the most pathetic point of my life, in fact, I may be at my most triumphant.

****

This last sentence is another one of those golden nuggets I wonder (looking back) how on earth I came up with given the shape I was in. But you can see pretty clearly from my observations that even in the brutal condition I was in, my mind was functioning at a pretty high level as far as maintaining a balanced viewpoint.

This level of sanity and reason and hope and spirit is what I hope for you too. It really can be a huge opportunity for you to fuse your personal sense of reason and hope. Reason and Hope are two ideas which are not usually uttered in the same sentence let alone logically applied with practical, measurable results.   Recognizing and accurately assessing a situation while at the same time seeing the probability of a positive outcome takes courage and practice. You will demonstrate, however, that not only is it <u>possible</u>, but it's the <u>only</u> really practical way to go!

iCanSir!

Journal Entries

_____
_____
_____
_____
_____
_____
_____
_____
_____
_____
_____
_____
_____
_____
_____
_____
_____
_____
_____
_____
_____
_____
_____
_____
_____

Day 12

"Keep your face to the sunshine and you cannot see the shadows."

Helen Keller

No Matter What!

Attitude is everything! As this quote from Helen Keller suggests, you see what you choose to see. In my training programs, I talk about a phenomenon known as Mr. Murphy of Murphy's Law fame. Do you recall Murphy's Law? "That which can go wrong, will go wrong."

O.K. so the order of the universe is such that we cannot control all of the 'stuff' that Old Man Murphy lays out before us. There's not much we can do about that. We simply can't control <u>all</u> of the variables in our lives. Thankfully, too. If we could, we'd go nuts trying to do so. As it is, some people drive themselves batty trying to control those few things they can. Anyhow, it's not news that we can't control everything that 'befalls' us at the hands of Mr. Murphy.

What may be news, however, is this: We can always control two variables. 1) The way we see it, and 2) the way we choose to act in response to it. How – in the first instance – we choose to perceive what we're confronted with will often be the most determinative factor in our success in tackling it. For example, if we see a challenge as insurmountable, it usually will be. When we look at a challenge and see it as doable, and then choose to respond by planning and acting in a step by step fashion to overcome it, our success is a practical certainty. Knowing this to be the case, it's hard to understand why we sometimes let ourselves, or those we care about, choose differently.

****

℞ iCanSir!

I am grateful for this glorious day. I took a sip of O.J. @ about 6 AM after waking up soaking in my sweat. As soon as I closed my eyes to the lovely slow sunrise of Albany, my face was warmed by a Zermatt[26] sunrise I had witnessed many times as a teenager. The sun was beautiful as it tipped the Matterhorn. I felt privileged to take part in it and I had. I sat there, or rather stood on my chalet's top floor balcony overlooking much of upper Zermatt, over the clay tile and slate rooftops upon which I had launched many eggs in the wee hours purely for my own homesick entertainment. I was taken back to one of those glorious sunrises with just a sip of ever so slightly outdated orange juice. Ironic the quote for the day! Eh?

1) Greater appreciation for each subsequent sunrise.
2) Renewed commitment to figuring out ways to make $$$ and travel.
3) Renewed commitment to balance.

****

Choose to see what lies ahead of you differently today. See it as a totally doable challenge. Choose now what you'll get out of this experience. Decide what lessons you'll learn, what difficulties you'll overcome, what rewards you'll reap, from this marathon.

How about those measurables? How about those intangibles?

Meditate. Take a few moments. As long as you need to. List 5 things you're truly grateful for today. No matter how small, concentrate on those things today.

---

[26] Zermatt is a tiny little town nestled in the southern Swiss Alps in the shadow of the Matterhorn. I had the great fortune of working there as a young man. I taught skiing and managed a small Chalet. Cooking and coaching: these are a few of my favorite things.

iCanSir!

Jot those outcomes and observations on today's Journal Page.

Journal Entries

_____

_____

_____

_____

_____

_____

_____

_____

_____

_____

_____

_____

_____

_____

_____

_____

_____

_____

_____

_____

Day 13

**"As simple as it sounds, we all must try to be the best person we can: by making the best choices, by making the most
of the talents we've been given."**

Mary Lou Retton

No Matter What!

When I first saw Mary Lou Retton take the stage at the Palace Theatre in Albany, New York, I was transfixed. Famed for her petit physique, her presence on stage was nothing short of gigantic!

Was it because she spoke so loudly? She didn't. Was it because she stood atop a riser or high heeled shoes? She didn't either. In fact, the diminutive Olympian wore flats!   Was it the 'jumbo-tron' image projected behind her above the stage? No, she was tiny even on that!

No, she was gigantic that day in upstate New York because as she shared her stories of her path to Olympic Gymnastic history, she beamed an energy of positivity and hope that was absolutely contagious!

Catch a new energy today. Then give it to someone else!

How often do you go through the day thinking - or at least hearing someone else think out loud – "It's one of those days!" in utter exasperation?

****

Maria and I went for a walk.

****

169

iCanSir!

Today, I had to let go of an old relationship again. (I say again because "once and for all" just doesn't do it. If you've had break ups in your life, you know what I mean.) It took a lot out of me. I know it doesn't seem like the best timing but you don't always exert total control over how and when people come in or out of your life. You can only control how you see it and how you act in response to it. I felt like I needed to deal with this today, of all days, for whatever reason. I needed to do a little mourning. Why not? I was mourning the temporary loss of my health and freedom of activity and financial independence, what's the harm in heaping an old relationship into the mix? Redemption starts with me and my responses!

****

1 deep breath. 2 deep breaths. I can handle anything! It's all good.

****

Take control of today and decide that one of <u>those</u> days is a day filled with joy and love and excitement and passion and hard work and fun! Then look into the mirror and say out loud:

"Yeeeeehaaaaah, it's one of <u>those</u> days!"

You know someone in your life right now who offers a healthy, vibrant energetic outlook that is genuinely refreshing and uplifting. It may even be you! Catch that spirit for yourself today. Call that person, ask the person over for a visit, speak with this person today. If it's you, meditate to tune into that side of you today. Catch the spirit. Get into it and let it get into you. Then give it away! Make sure someone else catches it too!

iCanSir!

Journal Entries

_____

_____

_____

_____

_____

_____

_____

_____

_____

_____

_____

_____

_____

_____

_____

_____

_____

_____

_____

_____

_____

_____

_____

_____

_____

_____

_____

Day 14

"We must always change, renew, rejuvenate ourselves; otherwise we harden."

Goethe

No Matter What!

Man alive! Goethe was amazing. You see even back a couple of hundred years ago, we knew that recreation was important.

Recreation.

Look at it literally. Re–Creation. At some point, man started doing a lot of things with an eye toward recreation. What was a day to day activity necessary for the maintenance of society, gradually became a recreational activity. A lot of activities might fit this category.

If it helps us change, renew and rejuvenate ourselves, it can be considered recreational. Whether you're doing it to compete, to stay fit, to meet men/women, to earn money, to live longer – what have you – if recreation is a key component, then it's probably good for you.

I needed to read this on this particular day because on this day I dealt with a recently failed relationship. It was a heavy day for me. I plowed through it but I needed to recreate something fierce.

****

Glorious day.

o.k., just that. My life needed to redeem itself. Literally. Re-Deem. I don't know really what deeming entails but I needed to do it again.

172

🎗 iCanSir!

How has cancer helped me begin to recreate?

1) Physically – I start from scratch, a clean slate of forgiven blood, guilt free lymphocytes and stress free organs. I replace old habits with new, healthy, productive, non-judgmental ones.
2) Mentally – My negativity is drastically subdued. I intend to keep it there.
3) Emotionally – I am regrouping in the center. I let go of a lot of anxiety.
4) Spiritually – Mom, God, the spirit, the energy, the universe, it runs through me. I connect. I'm certain of it.

My Hemoglobin is 9, White blood cell count is .4, platelets 24.

I feel great!

****

Today, ask yourself what will help you to "re-create". Jot your reflections onto today's Journal Page. "How is this experience helping me recreate physically, mentally, emotionally, spiritually, etc.?"

iCanSir!

Journal Entries

---

iCanSir!

Day 15

"I've always believed that you can think positive just as well as you can think negative."

Sugar Ray Robinson

No Matter What!

Like I've written before, it's a choice. The quality of your approach to your healing experience is a choice. The quality of your life's experience is a choice. The quality of your relationships is a choice.

You may not be used to this. You may be inclined – as many others are – to disagree with that philosophy. That's O.K. By the time you've practiced these skills and turned your cancer experience into a positive in your life you'll be a zealot! Ever hear the expression, "No zealot like the convert"? As an evangelist for the power of the subconscious mind, it's my job to "convert" you. Don't worry, though, I won't ask for donations or tithing, or for you to send me your first born anything, or take even one sip of anything you don't want to….Yet! (Juuuuuuust kidding!)

****

There are people in the world who will mock you in little ways to assure themselves that the way they're stuck in - the way they're scared to think themselves out of - is "the right one".

Don't allow these people to crawl into your head. They should be no more welcome there than a scorpion in a sleeping bag.

****

Again, I don't know where the whole scorpion thing came from but I love it! I'll give you a little background. From what I recall, about this time I'd been having some conversations with one of my team of doctors. I wasn't particularly impressed with this guy's attitude. He was a good man with good intentions, a wealth of experience but just not the best bed-side manner. He wasn't rude. He just wasn't tuned in to my enthusiasm, certainty or absolute requirement that only "positive" be spoken within my earshot. I had a talk with my team's leader about this requirement and from that point on – to my amazement – everyone's attitude improved! Amazing what kind of influence a little confidence can produce.

Ask yourself, "How did my emotions affect my healing today?"

_____

_____

_____

How's my body today?

_____

_____

_____

By now, can I get you to agree that what will get you across that finish line will be a combination effort of your body and your mind? If not, please turn to page 1 and re-read.

iCanSir!

Journal Entries

_____
_____
_____
_____
_____
_____
_____
_____
_____
_____
_____
_____
_____
_____
_____
_____
_____
_____
_____
_____
_____
_____
_____
_____

Day 16

"Take your work seriously,
but don't take yourself seriously."

Clint Eastwood

No Matter What!

The movies have the ability to inspire us to see things differently, to reach higher, to strive for more. Whether you like his acting style or not, you've got to recognize Clint Eastwood's talent. Beginning his film career as a cowboy, then as the movies' toughest cop as "Dirty" Harry Callahan, Eastwood's new pride is in directing and producing films. When asked what advice he would share with new actors or people in general, Eastwood delivered the quote at the top of the page.

Sometimes we all catch ourselves taking ourselves too seriously. When was the last time this happened to you? Take a moment to jot, on today's Journal Page, your thoughts on how taking yourself a little less seriously in certain areas of your life might help you to break down some barriers to what you're trying to accomplish.

****

Jan. 23 - I'm tired today (writing this on the 24th). Slept most of the 23rd. Didn't feel up to working or talking too much. Nice visit from the stylists[27] last night. Nice chat with one of the Patient Care Associates last night too. Sweetheart.

****

---

[27] A few months earlier I had worked with a hair salon's team of stylists and aestheticians. It had been a long term coaching project and we all became good friends as we worked together to figure out creative ways to enhance sales and team esprit de corps. I was floored when they all walked into my hospital room.

iCanSir!

Just as Clint Eastwood's desire to not take himself too seriously, allowed him to push his personal and professional boundaries, the same strategy can work for any of us. Today, be mindful of those things in your life you might take less seriously without abandoning your responsibility to them.

_____

_____

Enjoy today. Just relax and enjoy today!

𝄞iCanSir!

Journal Entries

_____

_____

_____

_____

_____

_____

_____

_____

_____

_____

_____

_____

_____

_____

_____

_____

_____

_____

_____

_____

Day 17

"It ain't over till it's over."

Yogi Berra

No Matter What!

'Nuff said!

Continuing with the Hollywood theme, think about some of the movies you've seen that have inspired you. List them on the lines below. Next to each title, write some thoughts about what message each film left you with.

_____

_____

_____

_____

_____

Make a plan to rent or borrow or purchase and <u>watch</u> these titles over the next several weeks as you recruit your mind to help in the work toward your recovery.

If it helps, here are some of my favorites:

Remember the Titans, Any Given Sunday, Scarface, Breaking Away, Chariots of Fire, Gallipoli, The Count of Monte Cristo, The Mighty Ducks, The Bad News Bears, Billy Elliot, Whale Rider, School of Rock, Marathon Man, The Abyss, It's a Wonderful Life, 12 O'Clock High, The Godfather - Parts I & II, My Left Foot, Singing in the Rain, A Bridge Too Far, The Great Escape, Ferris Bueller's Day Off, The

iCanSir!

Full Monty, Varsity Blues, The Shawshank Redemption, In the Name of the Father, To Kill a Mockingbird, The Hot Rock, Butch Cassidy & the Sundance Kid, Willy Wonka & the Chocolate Factory, What the Bleep Do We Know?, Goodfellas, Good Will Hunting, The Dish, The Sting, Akilah & the Bee, Freedom Writers and I Heart Huckabees.

Remember, these films don't have to be about anything in particular, as long as they inspire you for whatever reason!

I recall making the observation on this day that, letting go, detaching from the outcome of a particular effort, is an important step. I think it frees up a lot of resources to enable you to move on from a particular point. I felt a lot of pain and frustration as a result of a recent failed relationship. On this day I let it go again. When I really meditated on the idea of letting go and moving on, I noticed a real sense of lightening. I no longer carried a certain weight around. It was like the exercise when I forgave myself and my cancer. It was as though an enormous weight had been lifted from my burden.

Remember, you can't climb to the next level if you're not willing to let go of the level you're at now. Climbing a ladder requires you let go of one rung in order to reach for the next. In life, unfortunately we can't always see the next rung. It's there though.

What are your burdens? Are you still carrying yours? What needs to happen in order for you to loosen your grip? What outcomes are you holding on to? How is that helping you? What is that grip preventing you from reaching for now?

iCanSir!

Journal Entries

_____
_____
_____
_____
_____
_____
_____
_____
_____
_____
_____
_____
_____
_____
_____
_____
_____
_____
_____
_____
_____
_____
_____
_____

Day 18

"I never had to cheat. I get 'em with what I got."
Dave Winfield

No Matter What!

You're going to earn your stripes the best way...the hard way! As you pass each milestone in your recovery, make it through each day, reflecting as you go, you're accumulating credits on your transcript at the school of hard knocks. "F.U." as an old friend of mind used to call it. Whatever you call it, in the real world, these are the most valuable credits you can earn. That's why they are often the most expensive. With all this, there are a lot of shortcuts in this world. "A whole lot of cheatin' goin' on" as Jerry Lee Lewis might have sung.

But shortcuts are not what's going to get you well again. The psychological principles you're employing will make whatever treatment you're undergoing more effective and perhaps a little easier, but it's no short cut. Take some pride in that!

The exciting news is that there is no way you're going to go through this, and learn and apply these principles, without enjoying their benefits. Not only will you notice the benefits manifesting themselves in your physical health, but in every area of your life!

Just to give you an idea. At this point in my hospitalization my hemoglobin is now 10.6 (remember it was 4.0 when I was admitted), my hematocrit was 30.8, platelets 46 and Absolute Neutrophil Count (ANC) .8. Point of reference: my ANC had to be at least 1.0 in order for me to leave the hospital, 2.0 in order to have visitors in my home, 3.0 to be out and about with regularity and 4.0 might be considered normal.

ℛiCanSir!

Journal Entries

_____
_____
_____
_____
_____
_____
_____
_____
_____
_____
_____
_____
_____
_____
_____
_____
_____
_____
_____
_____
_____
_____
_____
_____

Day 19

"Te koura unuhanga roa."

Maori proverb

No Matter What!

Literally, "the long drawing out of the crayfish." The native tribes of New Zealand, the Maori, discovered that crayfish – a Kiwi dietary staple – are caught by drawing them out of their hideouts slowly. The Maori say this means that warriors can be defeated by tenacity as well as might. Even those of us who don't live on "the land of the long white cloud" can apply this to any endeavor. Your experience is no different. One step at a time, one day at a time, one page at a time, your mind/body partnership strengthens. One minute at a time, one heartbeat at a time, one concept at a time, you'll develop the skills you'll need, No Matter What!

This is one of those pages that I just couldn't bring myself to rewrite that much at all. The parallel to what we suffer during treatment for cancer is just too close. I remember finding it a simple step to get my head around the running metaphor. While I lay doubled-over in my bed suffering with nausea and all manner of unpleasant side effects and wondering how long it would take, the message in this page rang in my ears. "It won't last forever" I kept telling myself. "It might last a month. Hell I can stand on my head for a month." I kept reassuring myself. Read it as I wrote it for the runners. I think you'll get the point.

Contemplate the role that tenacity will play in your success. You may or may not be concerned with your finishing time. Either way, this race will have a particular time limit. For the sake of making this point, indulge me and let's say that the outer limit for you will be 5 hours. If it's longer, that's fine. I remember reading that it took over 28 hours for one woman to finish the NYC marathon… on crutches!

If that doesn't exemplify the spirit we're trying to match here, I don't know what could.

Anyhow, let's say 5 hours. What you're embarking on, will – at the outside – take you 5 hours. What you'll have to suffer through will last – at the most – 5 hours. At best, you'll zip through this in a personal best time. At worst, however, what you'll have to endure will only last 5 hours. Can you endure pain for 5 hours?[28] The answer to this – of course – is a resounding "YES"!

****

Impatient to get home. Where's my gratitude? I pause, I breathe in gratitude and exhale forgiveness.

I listen to Decaffeinated for like the 5th time since I've been here (23 days now). I contemplate a comment my nurse said last night after I mentioned that I don't really watch too much T.V. ordinarily. She said we only have 1400 waking minutes a day. Let's see. 16 waking hours considering 8 hours sleep. 16 x 60 = 960 by my calculations. Less than a thousand minutes a day!!

If that doesn't give you a sense of urgency. What – gold records, great times with kids, travel, $$$, grandkids, healthy, gratitude, love. Why – peace, balance, legacy.

****

Once you acknowledge that you really are tough as nails, the question then becomes "For what?" For what are you willing to endure that downside? On today's Journal Page, write all of the reasons you'll be

---

[28]If you've ever given birth to a child, you automatically get a gold star and must answer a screaming loud "YES" to this question!

willing to suffer whatever could befall you during those 5 potential hours. Write everything you'll get out of doing it. In this marathon – as in life – the "WHAT" is important…but not nearly as important as the "WHY"!

iCanSir!

Journal Entries

_____
_____
_____
_____
_____
_____
_____
_____
_____
_____
_____
_____
_____
_____
_____
_____
_____
_____
_____
_____
_____
_____
_____
_____

Day 20

"Push yourself again and again...Don't give an inch until the final buzzer sounds."

Larry Bird

No Matter What!

The idea of pushing yourself beyond what you "normally" can handle – I'm sure – is not a foreign one to you. In my most recent experience, survivors[29] have a pretty keen sense of what this means. Your treatment, how you handle yourself from now on, and working through this book, all will help you in two ways regarding the idea of pushing your boundaries.

1) You will expand your personal boundaries. That place on the map where you'll feel like quitting will be farther along the route than it was when you began this horrible, wonderful, paradoxical experience.

2) If ever you do get to that place where you feel like quitting, you will be mindful of an entirely new set of tools, resources you'll have within you, to push past that spot.

Today, be mindful of what type of information you find discouraging. Jot those thoughts and ideas on today's Journal Page.

_____
_____
_____

_____

[29] And by "survivor" – by the way – I certainly, absolutely, unequivocally and without ambiguity include patients AND caregivers, after diagnosis, during treatment and after remission! The whole crew. Survivors all!

190

Next, be mindful of how you might eliminate those types of ideas and reduce their impact on your thoughts.   Jot those thoughts as well. Finally, be mindful of strategies you might employ – ideas you might entertain – in order to be encouraged, inspired or motivated in response to some of that negative energy.   Jot your thoughts on that too.

_____
_____
_____

You'll employ this last set of ideas to actually replace potentially discouraging ideas with nurturing ones when you need them most!

****

Gratitude/forgiveness

I'm out of here today. Jim B. picked me up @ AMC today. I gave myself my neupagen shot sub-q and out we went.

As soon as we got to the parking garage the cold wind blew through the open walls of the parking garage and – although I wore a mask – the crisp cold fresh air was intoxicating. I stopped in my tracks and just breathed.

I came home, napped, went for a walk with Peter and Tessa. We stopped at Elaine and Mark's. Sammy had just made cookies. Mmmm. We didn't go inside. Just said hi.

Maria went to get my scrips filled.

I so missed just kidding around with the kids. My home feels enormous.

iCanSir!

Resentment for me is possibly the most debilitating.
Forgiveness and gratitude is the key (sic).

****

I remember feeling overwhelmed that my home was suddenly not my tiny hospital room anymore. I felt puny in my now huge house. If you could see our tiny little house, you'd appreciate the real irony of that. The funny thing here is that even in the joy of returning home, I still had to constantly fight back those creeping feelings of resentment, defeat and fear that inevitably become a part of our daily existence when cancer enters our lives. Mortality knocks once and forever the sound echoes. It makes it all the more important for us to be constantly mindful or our own courage. It makes it all the more important for us to be vigilant in constantly recognizing the hell we've walked through and survived!

iCanSir!

Journal Entries

_____
_____
_____
_____
_____
_____
_____
_____
_____
_____
_____
_____
_____
_____
_____
_____
_____
_____
_____
_____
_____
_____
_____
_____
_____

Day 21

**"Courage is not the absence of fear.
Courage is action in the presence of fear."**
Samuel Langhorn Clemens

No Matter What!

This quote by Mark Twain is absolutely one of my favorites. Today, think about your heroes. What makes them your heroes? When you really think about it, they're probably not your heroes because they lacked fear. They're probably your heroes because they did something – anything – probably in the face of danger. Danger can mean risk of any kind. It could mean the risk of losing money, losing social standing with peers, losing love, even the risk of physical pain, harm or death.

Who are your heroes?

_____

_____

What did your heroes do?

_____

_____

What risks did they face to do it?

_____

_____

In what ways can you consider what you do each day heroic?

_____

_____

Heroic to whom?

_____

Behave today as though you were wearing a cape!   Whenever you have a choice to make today, first ask yourself "what would my hero do?"

Then do exactly that.

No self respecting superhero goes by their lay person's formal name. What would your personal super-hero persona's nick name be?

_____

****

Second quote of the day…"Easy does it".

I drove to the doctor's office today and on the way home thought I was going to pass out. Not a good idea.

My body still needs a lot of rest.

****

Remember, I want you to "think" like the hero we both know you're capable of being. That doesn't mean I expect you to "do" everything you'd expect your hero to do. If you're supposed to be getting lots of rest, get the rest! If your hero would be getting lots of stuff done, then leverage yourself and get someone else to "do" the "doing" while you rest. Walt Disney "created" Disney World on the ceiling of his hospital room! He didn't dig the dirt himself you know! Would anyone accuse old Walt of not being a hero just because thousands of people did the "doing"? I don't think so.

Remember those measurables and non-measurables. What do you think? Is gratitude becoming a larger part of your response? Is it

iCanSir!

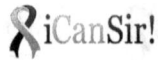

becoming a larger part of your mindfulness? What five things make your list today? Why? Are they different than the 5 things a week ago? Why do you suppose that's so?

Your mind can be the most powerful part of you while you're recovering and otherwise working on healing your body. Your mind. Your soul. The best parts of you, really. Remember our mantra.

No matter what happens to my body, my soul will always be perfect!
No Matter What!

iCanSir!

Journal Entries

_____
_____
_____
_____
_____
_____
_____
_____
_____
_____
_____
_____
_____
_____
_____
_____
_____
_____
_____
_____
_____
_____

iCanSir!

Journal Entries

_____
_____
_____
_____
_____
_____
_____
_____
_____
_____
_____
_____
_____
_____
_____
_____
_____
_____
_____
_____
_____
_____

Chapter Twelve
Quantum Physics and Marathon Running

I was incredulous.   It had been less than six months after my diagnosis, just 4 and a half months after the end of my first chemotherapeutic regimen, just moments after my third bone marrow biopsy, when Dr. Burkart   declared me "cancer-free".   It was an amazing day. I have to admit, however, that it was a day laced with a bit of denial.   I mean, I had dived headlong into my treatment and embraced my healing with such vigor and determination. As certain as I was in that, I have to admit that it was hard to believe that it had worked.

I believed in it. I really did. Maybe a part of me, however, wanted to be prepared to save face just in case. It was that part of me that I was wrestling with on that day.   The little devil on my shoulder saying things like, "don't get too excited, it might not really be true."

I guess it's normal to hear that voice.   It's normal to listen and somehow be attracted to that negative voice. It's normal to think first of the death and negativity and the outcomes we don't really want. Maybe deep down inside each of us there's a little bit of nihilist that secretly – and again, normally – has accepted our death and couldn't care less whether we live or die. I guess there's a certain attraction to being able to just give up. No more bills to pay, taxes to file, debts to worry about, neighbors to despise, envy to harbor, grudges to hold, friends to betray us, hard work to do, and every other silly thing that we let crawl deep into us and begin rusting ourselves from the inside out.

It would be so easy, and yes maybe normal, to just let go.

But you know what? To hell with normal!

I'd rather leave a legacy of triumph. If not over the actual obstacles themselves at least triumph over the fear of not making it past them.

This is the thing. After 180 days or so of discipline, isolation, nausea, loneliness, peppered with triumphant moments of gratitude, joy and even grace, I was out of the woods. Now what?

Being out of work for six months wrecked my financial situation. My private disability insurance had lapsed just weeks before my diagnosis and only thanks to a diligent insurance agent was my policy still in effect. The bottom line, however, was that my law practice and consulting business had completely dried up. The invoices kept coming, however, and my debt was becoming overwhelming. It was so bad, my bills had bills!

So what next?

It was so easy at that point to quickly become overwhelmed at the thought of recovering from this situation. My chemotherapy and recovery seemed like a pleasant distraction compared to the actual physical and mental work that was required of me now. It was crunch time and I had to figure out how to dig myself out of this hole that leukemia had put me in.

I know from years of paying attention that what you think about constantly begins to manifest itself in your life relatively quickly. I couldn't shake my consuming fear of overwhelming debt. It got worse and worse.

I'm telling you this because I want you to know the fears you feel, the nightmares you may have, the concern you may express to yourself and your loved ones about your financial situation when stuff like this happens, don't make you weak. They make you human.

The key at this point is to manage those fears into submission. The key at this point is to turn that energy into inspiration. The key at this point is to convert the paralyzing emotion of fear into action, courage and tenacity. Now it's time to buck up, re-acknowledge that this situation is here for a reason and plow through it. One step at a time!

I found that what helped me was a firm belief that I was surviving for a reason. It was valuable for me to recognize that there was absolutely no purpose in my surviving what I had been through only to file bankruptcy and fade away into obscurity. I deeply, deeply believe that just wasn't what was meant to be.

Again, I did a lot of meditating. I do it to this day. Looking back, I even wish I had done more of it! What I uncovered during this round of digging and sweeping was that I do have an idea of what my purpose is. I do know what it is that I was put here for. At least for now. I have an idea of what the highest best use of my time is.

I may be wrong. I often am. But for right now, spreading the word about what cancer patients and survivors and caregivers go through is important to me and I believe serves an important purpose.

Exactly HOW to accomplish this, I had no idea. It took me two years to figure it out and I'm still not sure I've got the perfect system but I haven't given up. I don't want you to either.

At first I ignored the "low hanging fruit" of my law practice and sought every possible way to avoid being a lawyer again. I swore I wouldn't thumb my nose at the universe by doing something I didn't LOVE "just to pay the bills". I swore I'd go full tilt into my speaking and writing so that I could live the life I'd been dreaming about for nearly a dozen years.

It's a nice idea. One that I absolutely, positively will NOT give up on. At the same time, it is not an idea that bore fruit right away. That dream would take a bit of time. The cancer organizations weren't exactly beating a path to my door. The bottom line was that I would NEED to do something to generate money to pay the bills, keep my house, feed my kids (not in that order).

ℛ iCanSir!

I tried working at the airport for barely above minimum wage.[30] If you recall I had run into my old high school mate who worked for the airline. I was so intrigued by the idea of traveling for "free" I thought it would be great. I also thought it would be a great way to get back in shape after being so sessile for so long. Work out, travel with the kids, make a little money at the same time. Sounds cool. Where do I sign up?

It actually served a wonderful purpose. While not really getting me any closer to working out my financial problems, as I regained my strength and confidence I was able to travel a little bit with my kids without costing me cash. I traded my sweat and time for a little money and whole lot of great memories and that itself was a great lesson for me.

After a great trip to Seattle with the kids to visit my sister, brother-in-law, niece and nephew, and a couple of flights to Atlanta to visit my buddy Stephen B. for lunch it was time to get real. I had to get a job. A real job. I needed something to pay the mortgage with until I figured out how I was going to make my living doing what I dreamed of. Writing and speaking.

The universe brings things to you when you're really in the zone. I made the decision to find something steady. A real job. It would be the first time I wasn't self employed since just after law school and this was weird for me. But, I had decided to do it and that was that. It was the right thing to do and I just had to do it.

I was networking in downtown Albany one afternoon. I stopped in to see my friend Roberto at his custom clothing store and update him on

---

[30] I love comic Chris Rock's idea of what the term "minimum wage" means. He says when a company offers minimum wage what they're really saying is "we'd like to pay you less, but the government won't let us." What's most funny to us is often so because it's so very true!

my new plan. Two minutes into the conversation, my friend Jeff walked by on the sidewalk.   Jeff was the Executive Director of a beautiful and historic 75 year-old theatre in Albany where we had presented Rock2Rebuild, the tsunami relief concert. Jeff told me that he had just been offered his dream job. He was going to take the helm at the Albany Ronald MacDonald House, a wonderful charity dedicated to helping families dealing with serious illness and hospitalization. Jeff and his family had been clients and real believers in the mission. This was one job Jeff could not turn down!

After the congratulations and all that, Jeff suggested that I seek his job as E.D. of the Theatre.   My concert promotion experience, my law degree, my marketing background and my positive relationship with City Hall would make me a shoe in.   Or so he thought.   He encouraged me to throw my hat in the ring and promised that his recommendation upon leaving would be that I take over.

I had a new short-term mission.   Deep down inside (and I felt this physically) I thought that maybe I was sacrificing something. I felt that maybe I was giving up independence, giving up a lifestyle, giving up on a dream. At the same time, that stack of bills was getting taller and taller.   So I ignored the stomachaches and went for it with everything I had.

I networked like a lunatic.   I talked to board members, friends and family of board members. I talked to the Mayor, I talked to influential business leaders. I was a maniac. I got an interview with the search committee.

The group who ran the theatre were really a group of successful, well intended business people who were a bit on the control freak side and had absolutely no idea how to keep creative people motivated. It's not their fault. I should have known better than to think that a completely attention deficit creative like myself and a group of type A conservatives would get along. I was relying on my charm and ability to wow them with my enthusiasm for the mission of creating the next generation of arts patrons. I should have realized that this was to be a marriage – or at least affair - made, if in not hell, at least in purgatory.

I didn't get the job. The vice chair called me into his office after 3 months of interviewing and follow up and then being ignored. He said that they had to hire someone else for the top job but they'd like me to be involved if I could handle being the number two guy.

I envisioned my pile of bills, thought about my kids, got my ego out of the way, ignored the pit in my stomach and said yes. I had to do what I had to do.

Another three months later, I met with the new E.D. Another three months after that, I started. It was a disaster from the get go and I should have seen it. I was so fixated on a steady paycheck that I completely ignored all of the signs that were screaming at me that this was NOT a good fit. Every step of the way my efforts to raise money were thwarted by the board. Promises made to me by the Mayor's office, and others, to help me woo important patrons were broken left and right. I had put myself in a position of relying on these people and they just weren't willing to put their energy (or their money) where their mouths were. My desire to do "the right thing" had clouded my vision, my judgment. I had convinced myself that in order to do the right thing I had to subrogate my dreams and aspirations or at least shroud them temporarily. It got me nowhere.

After 13 months of swallowing my pride, and beating my head against the wall, they fired me. I had failed miserably. Don't get me wrong. I raised a lot of money and brought in a lot of people who never would have had anything to do with the Theatre. Compared to the goals I had set for myself, however, I fell far below what I had set out to accomplish. I learned a lot about people though. Basically, however, thank God that was over!

I felt like a pound puppy just waiting to be put out of my misery. I didn't have the guts to quit.

iCanSir!

I kept telling myself it was because I needed the money.

I'm telling you this as a cautionary tale. I know that money is something we need to survive in our world. I like having money. Hell, I love having money. Although money doesn't buy happiness, I certainly know it makes for a hell of a down payment. At the same time, there are lots of ways to make money.

I sacrificed some of my dearest principles - independence, working from home, answering to only myself - to take that job. I ignored some profound instincts to take that job. Some of the people I answered to appeared to believe in very little of what I believe. I chose this under the guise of feeding my kids.

Did I do the right thing?

Who knows. I'm sure I'll sort all of that out over the next several years. I think that it was the right thing to do mostly because of the amazing experiences that I was able to take part in and the amazing people I was able to meet through my association with the Theatre. I certainly made the best of it. Although I could fill a whole book with stories and lessons from that year, I'll suffice it to say here that I made some great friends in the staff of the Theatre with whom I stay in touch and enjoy good times to this day. I met some amazing people and as a result of having a steady paycheck, I was able to take part in some things that "normal" people get to do.

One of these things was to have the extra time in the evenings and some weekends to begin to become involved in the Leukemia and Lymphoma Society's Team in Training Program. I'll close this book with a couple of stories from my association with the LLS and TNT. They highlight the point of sticking with your dream, no matter how circuitous the route that your dream takes you. You absolutely must continue keeping the end goal, the dream, in mind the entire time!

iCanSir!

As I mentioned earlier, I wrote my first book for a client of mine who was preparing to run in the New York City Marathon. *Jumper Cables for the Marathon Runner's Soul* is the book that I used during my treatment and is the book that provided the foundation for this book.

Back while I was writing the book I became aware of a program through which the LLS trains tens of thousands of marathon runners a year. Upon my recovery about a year later, I thought that the TNT program, as it's called, would make a great affiliation for my book. With my leukemia experience and my speaking ability, I thought that I should be working with the LLS to figure out a way to get my message into their runners' hands.

I approached the Executive Director of the LLS office in Albany. I had done some speaking for the LLS already as a survivor and explained my idea of getting my book into TNT participants' hands. The more I found out about the program the more I believed it was a perfect fit. I offered to re-write the book just for TNT and offered to share half the proceeds of any sales of the new book with the LLS. The local people liked the idea in principal and agreed to share the idea with the national office. They suggested that it would be an awesome idea if I participated in TNT and actually ran a marathon.

The idea of running 26.2 miles for any reason other than getting away from a really fit bear intent on eating me didn't appeal to me. The proposal made sense though. My pitch to the LLS would make a lot more sense if I had actually done the thing. I agreed and signed up. The object was to raise about $4000 for the LLS, train for and complete the marathon and do some speaking about the experience to other's interested in taking on the TNT challenge.

I went at it with gusto. I told all my friends and in a matter of weeks I accomplished the fund raising goal of $4000.00 having put about $1000.00 of my own money up for seed money. The challenge was to prove the value of my own material, train for the darn marathon and finish!

ℛ iCanSir!

It was fall of 2006. My marathon event for TNT was scheduled for January. The RockNRoll Arizona Marathon in Phoenix. I laid out a training program and overlaid it on top of my training book's 75 day motivational program. It fit like a glove and I was ready.

I began my training and stuck with it. About three weeks before my race in January, I was heading out for one of my last long runs before the race. I was to run about 17 miles on this Sunday and then taper down over the remaining two weeks before the race. About five miles into the run my knees completely gave out on me. The pain I felt was unbearable. It was joint pain so I knew better than to push myself through it. I ended up walking about 4 miles home and didn't get my long run in. I rested up for the race and hoped my knees would cooperate on race day.

In those last 2 weeks before the race, whenever I got anxious about my knees I would put it out of my mind. I'd say to myself "my knees are strong and healthy" and try not to think about it beyond that.

After the race I sent an email to my supporters. It tells the story nicely and I'll share excerpts of it with you here.

****

...I finished! My initial goal (this having been my very first marathon and first long distance run since I was a teenage runner) was simply to finish this race by hook or by crook! As many of you know, I was fully prepared to crawl across the finish line, if necessary. I went to AZ to prove only one thing, that leukemia doesn't have to stop us in our tracks!

℞ iCanSir!

. . .

Well, when I got to AZ and started hanging
out with the likes of other first timers as
well as experienced runners, I began to think
about other potential outcomes. I found out
that in order to be an "official finisher" I
would need to complete the 26.2 mile course -
in what I thought would be sweltering heat -
in under 7 hours. So 7 hours then became my
secondary objective!

Then I thought, "well, one ought to have a
real pie in the sky goal", ya know? Just in
case the God Mercury shone favorably upon me.
I figured, "boy, will I be just totally
psyched if I could break 6 hours!" I know,
crazy right?

I read the last pages of my Jumper Cables
book (crazy that I wrote that 5 years ago
before I ever even dreamed I would run a
marathon!) and got myself pumped up for the
challenge!

Well, at the start, it turned out to be 37
degrees. Bloody cold! I reached back to my
old days of standing atop Stratton Mountain
in my racing skins freezing my ass off in the
blistering wind, wrapped up in garbage bags
just trying to keep my thighs warm to the
very last minute before the beep, beep, beep
when I would "break the wand" and head down
the Giant Slalom course. Brrrrrr.

⸸ iCanSir!

Well that training (and being an upstater (no flatlander)) came in handy I tell you. I wrapped myself in baggies (picture to follow at some point I promise...) and we readied ourselves to strip down at the last possible minute before the start.

7:40 AM and off we went. Cccccccold. Mile 1 - 5. Not so much fun but I was beginning to warm up and the crowd was awesome. Reading my shirt which read "SURVIVOR" across the bottom in big letters, the crowd and other runners were very supportive! Runners were coming up next to me, hugging and high five-ing me, thanking me for inspiring them. "You go survivor!" they'd call out! "You go! You're awesome!" I'd reply! It made all the difference! The first five miles went by in an instant!

About mile 5 I started to feel great. I could run like that forever, I thought to myself (seriously knowing better deep inside). Miles 5-20 felt fantastic. I knew it wouldn't last the whole race, however, so I didn't let myself go too fast (fast, that's funny!). At mile 20, I was glad I had done that. At that point I figured "Hey, I'm going to break 7 hours!" I was psyched!

Mile 18. Hey, we could actually break 6 hours if we pick up the pace just a tiny bit! How cool is that! I ran into a deli on the course, grabbed three bags of potato chips (hey, you know me, I was starving!) for me and my running buddies! Hell, had I been

really ahead of schedule, I would have
stopped for a turkey sub. Don't laugh, I
heard that one lady on the half marathon
actually sat down in a McDonald's for
breakfast!

Mile 20-22 I began to become, let's say,
uncomfortable. My knees began really
hurting.

Mile 24, o.k. This sucks. My knees are
freaking killing me! What was I thinking?
But you know, hey, I'm actually having fun.
I can feel it!

Mile 25 Oh my God! My knees. I hope they
don't fall apart on me.

Mile 26 Wow, I'm almost there. God I hope
my legs don't fall off right now. My knees
are really killing me. I wonder if I'll die
when I cross the finish line?

The last two hundred yards. My running
buddy, Jenna, says "you wanna pour it on?" I
don't remember exactly what I said but I
remember thinking, "I honestly don't think I
have any more to pour on?" Seriously.
Afterwards when I asked about it, she
insisted that we began running just a little
faster toward the finish line but I'm still
dubious. We're still waiting for the video!
But, we did encourage each other those last
critical steps and I'm grateful for her being
there because honestly, I wanted to walk it
in at that point. I know, I know, Mr.

iCanSir!

Motivator wanted to walk? Well, hell yes I wanted to walk, my knees were killing me! Survivor, hello!? Don't I get to fall back on that? Tough crowd!

Hey, having come that far, and having had such a fantastic time of it, there was just no way I could walk across the finish line. Although, certainly to call what I did "running" would be a misappropriation of the word, I was going at a slightly faster pace than a walk, my knees were killing me, I had blisters on my toes and my whole body was aching (and hey, 23 months ago I had LEUKEMIA for crying out loud) I'm calling it RUNNING!

BUT SERIOUSLY, I reached down into the belly of my very soul, to all of the wonderful people who donated blood so I could live a few more weeks to take my chemotherapy, to the hard working scientists who had created Cladribine (the chemical that saved me), to the nurses, staffers and doctors who figured it all out and took such good care of me, to my wonderful family and friends who supported my positive attitude and nourished my soul with a lifetime of memories and love, to my children who have taught me everything!

I called out to these people a profound THANK YOU and reminded myself that just 23 months ago I crashed in a hospital bed, certain of my death, and now, right now, in this moment, I was about to cross the finish line of a 26.2 mile race...

℞ iCanSir!

... in less than 6 hours!

5 hours, 45 minutes, 5 seconds.

It's no record, certainly. BUT that finish line was in reality a new starting line for me. Another wonderful affirmation in a challenging life peppered about with good choices, decompensating episodes, epiphanies and a whole lot of wonderful people!

Thank you so very much for being a part of my life. I'm grateful to the universe for always managing to put me exactly where I need to be!

Here's to the next chapter. I wonder how it will read?!

Peace,

GPK

****

So. How will your next chapter read?   I know you may be thinking that you don't even know how this chapter will end. That's o.k. But it's good to have a goal. Something to shoot for. Something to reach for.

Think about what your next chapter will read like. Who might be in it? What might you do? What resources might you muster? What might you seek to accomplish in your next chapter? It's a blank page.

iCanSir!

It's up to you!

While I was in Phoenix I became aware of a series of running events presented by a company called Elite Racing. These events are all music related in that they feature bands throughout the races and the general themes of the events are all music related. If a participant finishes all six of these such events in one year, that participant is crowned "Rock Star". My goal for 2007 is to finish these six events. As of the writing of this book, since that first marathon, I've finished two more marathons. The Country Music Marathon in Nashville, Tennessee and the RockNRoll Marathon in San Diego, California. In the fall, my goal is to finish the remaining three events in the series. Three half-marathons on top of these three full-marathons and I will have run 117.9 miles to raise awareness for leukemia and cancer patients, caregivers and survivors.[31] I will be dubbed a "Rock Star" by the folks at Elite Racing. I thought it fitting!

Anyhow, my point is that this goal has brought awareness to my experience. I've been interviewed on every local network affiliate station in my hometown in Upstate New York since finishing that first marathon. I've raised the level of awareness for the work organizations like the LLS, the American Red Cross, and the American Cancer Society are doing to help people living with cancer. I've raised thousands of dollars for those organizations. I've been able to travel to extraordinary places and meet exceptional people. I've spoken to thousands of people and shared my story across the country.

Without really realizing it, perhaps, I've been fulfilling my purpose for the past ten months and loving each and every step of it. The pain the marathons have caused has long since been outweighed by the deep, deep sense of satisfaction that I've derived from helping people deal with their cancer experiences.

---

[31] I did finish the final three events in the Rock'N'Roll Series and was awarded the Rock Star medal. It was worth every ache, blister and pain!

ℛ iCanSir!

While I may still be practicing law to "pay the bills" I realize upon even the slightest reflection that the universe has brought to me the people and things I need to accomplish my purpose. I have managed to attract into my life the people and experiences I need to fulfill my deepest, truest mission. Quantum Physicists tell us that all matter and experience is energy. Different particles of energy vibrating at different frequencies manifesting themselves as experience to us, the observer.

Participating in our lives, actively manifesting our dreams in our conscious experience requires nothing more than mindfulness. Making decisions consistent with the "reality" we wish to experience draws nearer to us the energy in the universe that makes that reality possible. We vibrate at the frequency of stress and stress becomes manifest. We vibrate at the frequency of our dreams and … well you get the point.

I always believed in this stuff. Now I'm certain of it.

You can make manifest your dreams too. It may take time to experience that dream in your life but it takes but a moment to see that dream in your mind. The more often you see it in your mind, I'm convinced, the sooner you'll see it in your life.

If you had told me in the summer of 2006 that one year later I would have run and completed three marathons, raised thousands for research and spoken to thousands of people about the power of the human mind and the material I had been teaching for over a decade, would I have believed you? I would have believed it to be possible but, honestly, I may have been dubious that it would be me who did it.

Today I write these final words as a man who still struggles with certainty every day. I still wake up occasionally wondering if or when I'll have to deal with a relapse of my cancer. Wondering when and if my "Uncle Leu" will visit again as my kids and I jokingly refer to my leukemia.   I still worry about money and marketing my speaking services and finding law clients and, yes, paying the bills.   I am still mindful that I have expensive music college tuition to raise and a teenage daughter to get through high school with her self-esteem intact.   I still wonder about the decisions I've made while raising my kids.   I still hope that I've instilled in them the senses of certainty and confidence and compassion and interdependence that I hope they've grown into.   I still ponder those heavy questions.

I'm still a human becoming.   Just like you.

I ponder, however, knowing this: As a human becoming I need to make myself open to the rattle and hum of the universe.   Just like you.   As a human becoming I need to continue my emotional archaeology every day.   Digging and sweeping for the how's and why's of my life and how to improve the decisions that I make.   Just like you.   As a human becoming I need to embrace my condition of interdependence and relinquish my ego to follow the truest purpose that stirs within me.   Just like you!

Shhhhh.   Listen for it.   Hmmmmm.   Feel it.   Ahhhhh.   See it.   Your truest calling is there.   It may be cleverly disguised as hardship, confusion, discomfort.   It may even be disguised as cancer.   Find that inner purpose.   Get in tune with it.   Sync up with it.   You owe it to yourself.   You deserve it.   It is meant for you!

ℝ iCanSir!

APPENDIX A
"Doing" the lists!

Use this Appendix to create your lists and your statement of purpose. I strongly recommend you do this at least once a week for the first week when starting this program or restarting this program once you've found that life may have stepped in the way. Hey it happens! After that, do this once a week for a month. Then, do this once a month for the rest of your long, healthy, uncertain and adventurous life!

The purpose of these worksheets is to channel and focus your thinking toward the creation of a concise statement of what you were born to do. Your mission. Your Purpose! This process may be challenging, it may not be. It may require some serious deliberation, it may not. It may require painful introspection. It may cause you to realize those things which you've not yet done. It may cause you to breathe a sigh of relief. It may do all of these things. It may do none of them. What it will certainly do, however, is cause you to think about your life in a way most people simply never do. Most people go about their lives never having invested the time, the money, or the pain to discover, uncover or remember what's truly important to them, what noble purpose their life was meant to be invested in pursuing, and creating the habits necessary to make those dreams reality. This process, the Statement of Purpose, is one of many toward creating those habits!

Step One: Your lists!

The first step is to create a few lists which will channel your focus toward the goals, dreams and objectives which truly are important to you. The point is to identify those objectives that would fulfill your dreams when accomplished and the mere pursuit of which would fulfill your purpose. We accomplish this by creating three lists.

iCanSir!

Your Lottery List:

The first list is created by setting aside two minutes (no more or less at this stage), putting pen to paper and simply writing and writing until the time's up. What you'll write is a list of all of those things you would seek to accomplish over the next thirty years if you knew you could not fail. Following appears a sample list of many different dreams, goals and objectives that many clients have identified over the years. They're not meant to be YOUR goals or dreams, just ideas which may prompt your thinking along the lines of what you truly would like to pursue if you were mindful of the boundless resources that could be brought to bear toward creating your dreams. Use the two minutes to simply write. Do not judge or evaluate as you go. There will be plenty of time for this type of "reality check" as you create your dreams. If you need a bit of help with this – or any of the lists – see the sample lists that follow each section. Many times the first stumbling block to our really big dreams appears to be money (or the lack of it). This first list is therefore called the Lottery List because most folks can relate to the idea of hitting the lottery and all of their dreams coming true. It may have a bit of fantasy in it but it serves as a good starting point for identifying the things that put a smile on our face or light a spark in our heart. Set an egg timer at two minutes and write those things here…

LOTTERY LIST

Over the next thirty years, if I knew that I absolutely could not fail, these are the things I would seek to see, be, do and/or have…

_____
_____
_____
_____
_____
_____

_____

_____

_____

_____

_____

_____

_____

Your Lightning List:

The second list is created by setting aside two minutes to write all of those things you'd seek to see, be, do and/or have over the next three years IF 1) you absolutely knew you could not fail and 2) you knew that three years from today's date, you'd be struck by lightning and killed. In fact, at the top of this list, write today's date and then the same date three years from now. This will serve to punctuate for your subconscious mind that our time here is finite and that if we are to pursue our noble goals, there isn't time to waste! Set those two minutes on the clock again and write those things here…

LIGHTNING LIST

Today's Date: _____ (+ 3 years) = _____

Over the next three years, if I knew that I absolutely could not fail, these are the things I would seek to see, be, do and/or have…

_____

_____

_____

_____

_____

_____

_____

_____

_____

_____

_____

_____

_____

_____

_____

_____

_____

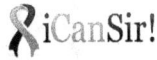

Your "Edge of the bed" List:

The third list is created by imagining the unimaginable. After reading this paragraph close your eyes for twenty seconds or so. Imagine, really imagine, what it would be like to find yourself in the hospital. Your doctors have told you that you are not likely to live past the end of the week. More importantly, imagine how it would feel to BELIEVE what the doctors were telling you. Imagine that they're right. I know this is hard, but imagine what that would be like. As you sit there on the edge of the bed, reflecting back on the past three months, what would you wish you had accomplished? To punctuate the timeline for you, write today's date and the date it was 90 days ago. What would you wish you had invested those precious 90 days doing? Set two minutes on the clock and write those things here...

EDGE OF THE BED LIST

Today's Date: _____ (- 90 days) = _____

What do I wish I'd invested my time with over these past 90 days?
What do I wish I'd seen, been, done and/or had these past 90 days?
What do I regret not having seen, been, done and/or had?

iCanSir!

_____
_____
_____
_____
_____
_____
_____
_____
_____
_____
_____
_____
_____
_____
_____

Simple Pleasures/Sample Goals[32]

Water ski in January   Snow ski in July
Rock Climb   Fire walk
Ride a Harley Davidson   Laugh with kids
Travel – Egypt, Canada, Venezuela, Rio, Antarctica, Cuba,
Switzerland, Australia, Japan, Alaska, Africa, China, Russia, India,
Chicago, Boston, London, L.A., New York City!
Ride the Orient Express   Wade in the ocean
Skydive off the Eiffel Tower   Plant a tree
Rafting   Cure cancer

_____

[32] This is a combined list of many goals that people have shared with me over the past decade of teaching this stuff in a seminar by the same title as this book. Interspersed throughout the list are items which some friends of mine and I added one day coming back from a water-ski trip. I hope they give you a little jump-start and remind you to DREAM BIG!

iCanSir!

Help someone with cancer

Make up a "There once was a man from ..." limericks

Fly a bi-plane upside down

Scuba dive

Seal a driveway

Parasail

Walk on the beach at midnight

Stare out at the ocean for 1 hour & just think

Duck hunt

Build a pillow fort

Ride a horse

Write a romantic love poem

Play Scrabble

Ride the Tower of Terror at Disney

Skateboard

Jet boating in New Zealand

Build a house

Get off school for a day to learn something elsewhere

Make a sandwich

Eat a box of strawberries

Be a great role model

Snowmobile

Get released from prison

Cliff diving

Drive fast through a city's downtown at midnight

Ride around the Washington D.C. monuments at night

Play paintball

Attend a corporate outing

Thank your parents

Hike the Appalachian Trail

Make a television commercial

Play with friends

Roller blade

Put a wreath on a grave

Ride a bike off a jump into a pool

Teach someone something

Fly in a Mig fighter

Wing walk

Snorkel in the Caymans

Jetski

Build a sandcastle

Make a model airplane

Skinny dip

Build an Igloo

Eat sushi

Ride a roller coaster w/some kids

Play Backgammon

Tubing

Ride a hot air balloon

Feed the hungry

Make some soup

Climb a tree

Snowboard

Horseback riding

Dive 3 meters

Act in a play

Tryout for a pro team

Thank a client

Thank God

Thank a Veteran

Go to a concert

Jump on a bike

Bowl

Eat ice cream

Meditate

Barefoot ski

iCanSir!

Talk yourself out of a speeding ticket   Drive a race car
Ride a 4 wheeler   Ride the space shuttle
Pole vault   Hire a maid
Ride in a limousine   Earn a black belt
Turn a cartwheel   Thank your kids
Sing a song   Cuddle with a dog or cat
Cuddle with your partner   Watch an old movie
Meditate for 24 hours straight   Fast for 4 days
Drink a milkshake   Shave your head
Rent a movie   Borrow a book
Write a screenplay about your life   Lend a book
Read a book   Read two books
Read to children   Thank your teachers
Have a disco party   Have any party
Have a new year's party…   in July
Throw a suitcase party   Throw a dinner party
Have 10 adults over and have a contest to see who can make the
yummiest frozen drinks
Knit a sweater   Build a lean-to
Eat an ice cream sundae   Climb a mountain
Take a leisurely hike   Swim in a river
Find a mentor   Find a mentee
Buy a police officer a fruit cup
(better for him/her than coffee and donuts)
Visit the VA hospital
…During the holidays
…Thank the Vets for their sacrifices
Tell someone you love him/her   or not
Take off your clothes and dance a jig   Take yourself for a walk
Smoke a cigar (don't inhale)   Bungee jump
Shoot a gun   Destroy a gun
Visit an aquarium
… a zoo
… a planetarium
… an animal shelter
Make love by moonlight   by firelight

in a car
Build a piece of furniture
Invite the neighbors over
... for dinner
... for lunch
... for breakfast
Call for a parent/teacher conference... for no specific reason
Be a mentor
Apologize to someone you've hurt
Go camping
Visit a shut-in
Play it cool
Roast a turkey
Make a map of your body's tickle spots
... give it to your partner
... to your kids
... to your employer
Make spaghetti sauce
Go window shopping
Make a deposit into your savings account
Run around your house 3 times
... shouting "ding dong the wicked witch is dead!"
Make a batch of cookies
Tell a child that there's something extra special about him/her
... then list ten things!

in a hot tub
a mailbox
Forgive yourself
Accept yourself

Jump in a hot spring
Say a prayer
Jump in a cold spring
Do a cross-word puzzle
Bounce on your bed
Go grocery shopping

Bake a pie
Buy some windows

Step Two: Your Building Blocks!

Next, you must identify the areas of your life that provide the many different degrees of satisfaction in your life. The areas among which you must balance your precious time. An easy way to do this is to identify the goals on your lists above which really provide the most "juice" for you. These are usually those items which end up on your 90-day (Edge of the Bed) list. Usually, but not always. It may help to circle on the lists above, those dreams which get you the most excited.

Those dreams, the pursuit of which would really give you unparalleled inspiration to live.

Once you identify these, think of a word that describes the role you play in pursuing it. For instance, if the goal on your list is to be a great husband or wife then "husband", "wife", "spouse" or "partner" could be words used to describe that "role". Sometimes, it helps to first categorize the dreams into discreet areas – or dimensions - of your life. Some people prefer to do this, others don't. It might help. If it doesn't, go ahead without first categorizing your dreams. It'll be fine! Either way, the point of the exercise is that you end up with a list of the Roles that you play in your life. The short lists of both sample Dimensions and Roles below may help you to pick words to describe these ideas.

The end result of this section will be to write onto the MASTER WORKSHEET page those Roles that you identify yourself playing in pursuit of your most important objectives, dreams and goals. You should write these Roles on the appropriate lines toward the top of the MASTER WORKSHEET next to the words "I am a/an" for each of the Dimensions set out on the left side of the page. For example:

Dimension	*Role*
Relationships/Family	*Father*

1) I am[33] a/an ___father___

Sample Dimensions

Career	Family	Physical
Spiritual	Inner	Social
Intellectual	Financial	Personal Desires
Environmental	_____	_____

_____

[33]Always articulate these in what I call the "successful tense", i.e.: I am rather than "I will be" or "I want to"…

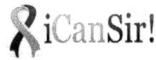

iCanSir!

Sample Roles

Business Builder	Mother/Father	Son/Daughter
Half-brother/sister	Sister/Brother	Step-sibling
Cousin	Uncle/Aunt	Provider
Partner	Evangelist	Friend
Supporter	Booster	Coach
Reporter	Employer	Artist
Performer	Trouble Shooter	Real Estate Agent
Mechanic	Athlete	Body builder
Individual	Lover	Caregiver
Teacher	Leader	Guide
Achiever	Bread winner	Builder
Networker	Salesperson	Journalist
Writer	Thrill seeker	Time manager
Task master	Ass kicker	Drill Sergeant
Answers person	Ideas person	Designer
Detail person	Planner	Organizer
Doer	Fund-raiser	Developer

Next, you're going to choose some modifying words to describe you at your best while playing that particular Role in your life. Some sample words can be found below. Combine your Roles and the modifying words corresponding to that Role and fill in the second section of the final worksheet. For example:

1) I am a/an __loving__ and _patient_ ___father___
               adj./adv.   adj./adv.   Role

Sample Adverbs/Adjectives

Highly	Uniquely	Passionately	Morally
Ethically	Creatively	Handily	Quickly

Effectively	Efficiently	Frugally	Totally
Superbly	With dispatch	Consistently	Devout
Persistent	Ambitious	Super-charged	Intelligent
Unreasonable	Talented	Focused	Exciting
Motivated	Patient	Enthusiastic	Articulate
Conscientious	Supportive	Nurturing	Passionate
Listening	Reaching	Inspiring	Constructive
Creative	Gentle	Crazy	Confident
Strong	Chiseled	Ethical	Generous
Gorgeous	Sexy	Shy	Physical
Ethereal	Inspired	Serious	Inspiring
Detail oriented	Well-versed	Committed	Balanced
Congenial	Friendly	Gregarious	Daring
Aggressive	Persistent	Consistent	Grateful
Affectionate	Independent	Honorable	Reliable
Punctual	Extraordinary	Inclined	Extreme
Calm	Balanced	Thoughtful	Reserved
Jocular	Hopeful	Tender	Tough

Next, you're going to choose some modifying words to describe what happens when you are at your best while playing that particular Role in your life. Who benefits, what benefits are created. What happens. When you come up with an idea, ask yourself "so what?" For example: Let's say I'm at my best as a father by being patient and loving. Who benefits from that? My children, right? So, my beneficiaries include my "children." Don't I benefit, doesn't my whole family benefit, doesn't my spouse or partner benefit from me being my best at that Role? So, my other beneficiaries might include, "myself", "my family", "my community". Continuously asking "so what?" gets you closer to the heart of the matter. For instance, when I'm at my best at being a dad, there is less shouting and anxiety around the house. "So what?" Less anxiety means more happiness, more focus on positive things. "So what?" More happiness means more stability, greater likelihood that the children will have confidence to pursue their dreams. "So what?" brings us to the point.

ℛiCanSir!

For example:

1) I _create_ _a stable and nurturing home_ for _my children_ and
　　action word　　　　benefit　　　　　　beneficiary1

myself , we all grow toward _greater confidence_ & _self-actualization_!
beneficiary2　　　　　　　　benefit　　　　　　　benefit

Take a crack at it.

_____

_____

_____

_____

_____

_____

_____

_____

_____

_____

_____

_____

_____

_____

_____

_____

_____

_____

_____

iCanSir!

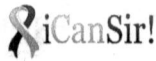

Sample Action Words

Add	Apply	Ask	Become
Begin	Build	Call	Carry
Change	Combine	Complete	Consider
Contact	Contribute	Convert	Create
Determine	Develop	Discover	Do
Eliminate	Enjoy	Enroll	Examine
File	Finance	Find out	Fix
Find	Formulate	Fashion	Forage
Get	Give	Generate	Go
Gather	Identify	Incorporate	Increase
Instruct	Insure	Invest	Join
Keep	Learn	Locate	Make
Maximize	Meet	Minimize	Move
Normalize	Obtain	Open	Operate
Overcome	Own	Participate	Pay
Prepare	Protect	Put	Qualify
Raise	Read	Reduce	Refinance
Remove	Replace	Respect	Select
Send	Show	Spend	Start
Stop	Store	Structure	Substitute
Take	Teach	Train	Turn
Upgrade	Undertake	Use	Utilize
Withdraw	Work	Write	Fix
Rearrange	Coach	Inspire	Know
Tell	Train	Satisfy	Announce
Devise	Mediate	Articulate	Excite
Meditate	Choose	Plan	Expedite
Cook	Prepare	Transport	Tune in

iCanSir!

Sample Benefits

Peace of mind	Security	Wealth
Great relationship	Fame	Maturity
Meaningful Career	Power	Happiness
Debt Reduction	Gratitude	Freedom
Good Health	Help others	Control
Meet Mr./Ms. "Right"	Balance	Closer to God
Greater Understanding	Travel	Respect
Relieve suffering	Retirement	Opportunity
Contributing time	Knowledge	Help
Overcoming Obstacles	Longevity	Independence
Material things	Lower blood pressure	
Greater Intimacy	Reduced dependency	
Sense of accomplishment	Love	_____

Sample Beneficiaries

Self	Spouse/Partner	Children
Family	Grandchildren	Friends
Loved ones	Co-workers	Employees
Customers	Patients	Suppliers
Downline/Upline	Clients	Company
Leaders	Fellow countrymen	Community

Finally, after each of these pairs of sentences, we add a sentence for the third 'B', Bottlenecks. Bottlenecks are areas in your life, that – if you made a change or improvement in – would dramatically impact your ability to achieve your goals. After each objective or role, identify the stumbling blocks or challenges that have prevented you from reaching this goal before.

For example: If one of my objectives is to be a great dad and I've identified the benefits that are created by that action and I've identified the beneficiaries of that goal as my children, then I add a third sentence to this set as follows:

iCanSir!

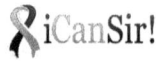

I project myself a year into the future and ask myself my bottleneck-identifying question, "In the past year, what stopped me from being a loving and patient father?" Two of the bottlenecks I identify by asking this question might be "impatience" and "yelling".

1) I continually work on *being more patient* and am particularly *careful to yell as infrequently as I possibly can."*

Sample Bottlenecks

Impatience	Intolerance	Intemperance
Short Temper	Bad Attitude	Ingratitude
Negative Thinking	Pessimism	Fearful
Poor self-image	Closing the sale	Prospecting
Pushy	Overbearing	Disrespectful
Insensitive	Selfish	Low compassion
Self-absorption	Undisciplined	Disorganized
Inflexible	Unstructured	Distrustful
Untrustworthy	Irresponsible	Dependent
Closed minded	Poor planning	Co-dependent
Excitable	Anxious	_____

Step Three: Your Statement of Purpose!

Continue working with these sentences until you've drafted a half dozen or so such sentences that accurately portray those things that are truly important to you. Remember, Shakespeare is quoted as having said that the secret to good writing is re-writing! This will seem rough at first. It may seem ridiculous. Believe me, hundreds of people have used this formula. They've identified and articulated a Statement of Purpose. Many of them felt silly at first. Many of them believed it would help, some of them didn't. But all of those people who put the effort into this exercise left with a profoundly greater sense of what they are truly meant to see, be, do and have in this life. This mindfulness is a first critical step toward creating the plans and habits by which we transform our dreams in our reality!

RECAP: By combining the three sentences which we've crafted for each Role and with a little tweaking here and there...

Family/Relationship - Father
> *I am a/an __father__*
> I am a/an _PATIENT_ and _LOVING_ _FATHER_
> I _create_ a stable and nurturing home _for_ _my children_ and _myself_, we all grow to*ward greater confidence and self- actualization*_!
> I continually work on *being more patient* and am particularly *careful to yell as infrequently as possible*."

Rough Draft (after just a bit of tweaking - turning some of the negative language into positive):

I am a patient and loving father. I create a stable and nurturing home for my children and myself and - as a result – we all grow toward greater confidence and self-actualization! I continually work on being more patient and am particularly careful to communicate calmly and patiently while gaining more and more control over my temper.

Imagine how powerful this will become as we add roles and continue to fine tune this!

iCanSir!

MASTER WORKSHEET

"The only true happiness comes from squandering ourselves for a purpose."

William Cowper

Roles - the "whats", what roles you play

Dimensions	**Roles**
Health/Personal	**1) I am a/an** _____
Relationships/Family	**2) I am a/an** _____
Professional/Financial	**3) I am a/an** _____
Spiritual/Emotional	**4) I am a/an** _____
Spiritual/Emotional	**5) I am a/an** _____

Adjectives/Adverbs - "the hows" of you being at your best in these roles

1) I am a/an _____ and _____ _____
           adj./adv.   adj./adv.   role

2) I am a/an _____ and _____ _____
           adj./adv.   adj./adv.   role

3) I am a/an _____ and _____ _____
           adj./adv.   adj./adv.   role

4) I am a/an _____ and _____ _____
           adj./adv.   adj./adv.   role

Benefits and Beneficiaries - "the whats and for whoms"

1) I _____ _____ for _____ and _____.
        action word   benefit   beneficiary   beneficiary2

2) I _____ _____ for _____ and _____.
        action word   benefit   beneficiary   beneficiary2

3) I _____ _____ for _____ and _____.
        action word   benefit   beneficiary   beneficiary2

4) I _____ _____ for _____ and _____.
        action word   benefit   beneficiary   beneficiary2

Bottlenecks - "the why nots"

1) I work to reduce _____ each day, which frees me to live my purpose!
                Bottleneck

Rewrite: Examine daily for 21 days, examine weekly forever!

With even just a little planning, every Goal consists of a finite series of tasks. Upon the completion of all of the tasks, the Goal has been achieved. More importantly, in pursuing the tasks you are fulfilled. Joy comes from the journey. What comes of the destination? A view to another Goal! Establishing a game plan - a relatively detailed "road map" of the various tasks associated with the accomplishment of the Goal - is a critical step in pursuing the Goal. A game plan is formed by brainstorming as many of the tasks as you can then think of, identifying all of the various means by which you can garner the support, assistance, information, contacts, etc. you'll need and stating the Goal in a positive manner.

> "I have six honest serving men, they taught me all I knew.
> They are What and Where and When,
> How and Why and Who!"
>
> Rudyard Kipling

Identify your six honest serving folk for each of the primary Goals in your life. Then articulate these statements in what I call the "successful tense". You've heard these sentences referred to as affirmations. I'll use "Who" for an example of an affirmation I might formulate if my Goal is to earn $10,000.00 more this year than last: "I am working with my clients/customers to provide a greater value to them this year and I am concentrating on increasing the number of referrals from them. In so providing a greater benefit, I am earning a greater reward. I am earning $XX,XXX in _____ (this year)." The keys to this affirmation are 1) "I am". I remind myself in the "successful tense." 2) I remind myself of the price I am willing to pay (greater contribution, more networking/referrals). 3) I remind myself of the specific reward (Goal) I seek.

Do this for each goal you consider important enough to make happen. Create the statement of purpose and then plan according to the six serving men/women. Break it down into doable, measurable tasks. Set to accomplishing those tasks as your time allows. Day by day, you gradually start performing more and more of the necessary tasks associated with living your dream. Day by day, you eventually begin creating the habits. Day by day, you begin to notice the effects of your discipline!

"Rrrrrrrepetition is the mother of education!"

Dr. VandenBerg, my 6th Grade German teacher

Affirmations, when written in the successful tense and read out loud at least twice a day (and as often as possible in between), have a profound impact on your attitude and how quickly you accomplish your <u>G</u>oal. God bless Dr. VandenBerg. How right he was!

In case there was any confusion…

"Rrrrrrrepetition is the mother of education!" (Ibid).

Once the goal is clear, once it's broken down, once the affirmation is written, it becomes a question of leaving it to your subconscious mind to come up with the how you're going to do it!

Your purpose will help drive you to it. So will courage. Just know this. Once you've clarified your goals, written them into your life, broken them down and created affirmations around them, you are better than halfway there! That's just the way the universe works! Keep in touch!

iCanSir!

Epilogue

A life of many!

Mine is a life of many. It's made up of and shared with a diverse
group of people, all with at least 2 things in common. First, a
commitment shared with me to live life vigorously. Second, a desire
to do so with the shared
blessings of many people.

I suffered a challenge which made me sleep.
When I opened my eyes, you all were there.

Join me in a celebration of our journey together and my gratitude for
you being part of my life. We need not wait for a cure in order to
celebrate. Life need not be health. Life, for us, simply can be.

Dance with me at our life's banquet. Sit with me at my table and let
us slurp the quantum soup and gnaw the cosmic offal. We'll tear
pieces off of the universal loaf and sop up the abundance…lest we
waste a drop!

Let us gulp it down and then howl our gratitude unto the mountains,
over the seas and up to the moon and the stars.

We'll yodel and yawp
'til the wolves lie sleeping at our feet!

iCanSir!

No matter what happens to our bodies, our souls will always be perfect!
No Matter What!

With Gratitude!
GPK

Library of Congress Catalog # pending

www.georgepkansas.com

ISBN 978-0-9763573-3-9 Hardcover
ISBN 978-0-9763573-4-6 Ebook
ISBN 978-0-9763573-5-3 Softcover

journeypress

9 780976 357353